A PLACE OF HEALING

A PLACE OF HEALING

Working with Nature & Soul at the End of Life

MICHAEL KEARNEY, M.D.

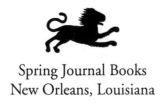

Spring Journal Books
New Orleans, Louisiana

Published by:
Spring Journal, Inc.
New Orleans, Louisiana USA
www.springjournalandbooks.com

Previously published as:
A Place of Healing: Working with Suffering in Living and Dying
Oxford, U.K.: Oxford University Press, 2000.

Publishing Support:
Northern Graphic Design & Publishing
info@ncarto.com
Cover design: Matt Schoen

Cover art: Nasturtiums with the Painting "Dance" (1912),
by Henri Matisse © The Metropolitan Museum of Art / Art
Resource, NY. Used with permission.

Text printed on acid-free paper

Library of Congress Cataloging-in-Publication Data Pending

This book is dedicated to the memory of my parents,

Ann Kinmonth and Kevin Kearney. From them both,

and from the lineage we share, I have received

example, curiosity, and a longing to know

more of the mystery of healing.

Contents

Foreword

Balfour Mount
Eric M. Flanders Professor of Palliative Medicine (retired),
McGill University, Montreal

Since the dawn of human development, people have known themselves to be something more than body and mind. Reality has been understood to involve a hierarchy of states of being that includes matter, body, soul and spirit.[1] The empirical, physical world has been seen as existing in community with complementary transcendent domains. It is, or perhaps more accurately, *was,* widely held that the soul and spirit may be experienced but not proven. They are variously conceived as having to do with healing, wholeness, immortality, connectedness, purpose, meaning, inner journey that involves the depth of our being and the potential for inner peace.

Modernity, that is, Western, post-Enlightenment society with its positivist stance, is the first major civilization to deny these premises. The staggering productivity of science during the past century has led to a shift in our assumptions about its role. No longer is science viewed as simply one way of learning about the nature of reality. Science has passed from "servant-tool" to supreme arbiter, defining what is "real." Furthermore, the marriage of scientific materialism and capitalism has enshrined a set of global values in the wake of which other ways of coming to know and understand the cosmos are dismissed—shrugged off as primitive vestiges of our psychic adolescence.

The total dismissal of the spiritual domain is now so widely accepted that we may lose sight of how recent this shift has been. Freud, who died in 1939, once declared, "Humanity has always known it possesses a spirit; it was my task to show that it has instincts as well." In commenting on this statement, psychiatrist Viktor Frankl observed, "I myself feel that humanity has demonstrated *ad nauseam* in recent years that it has instincts, drives. Today it appears more important to remind man that

---

[1] Ken Wilber, *The Marriage of Sense and Soul: Integrating Science and Religion* (New York: Random House, 1998).

he has a spirit, that he is a spiritual being."[2] Frankl went on to say, "Man lives in three dimensions: the somatic, the mental and the spiritual. The spiritual dimension cannot be ignored, for it is what makes us human."[3]

How do we understand such a claim in a secular age? In 1987 *Palliative Medicine*, with its self-proclaimed concern for the body, mind and spirit, was recognized as a new medical specialty in the United Kingdom. Indeed, the World Health Organization included "control of spiritual problems" in its 1990 definition of palliative care.[4]

By 1992, however, Michael Kearney predicted that the holistic focus of the new discipline might be lost under the weight of the biomedical model. He feared that consideration of the whole person would be replaced by a narrower focus that was limited to concern for physical symptoms; in short, that the new specialists would be reduced to "symptomatologists."[5] His words appear to have been prophetic. In 1997 a leading academic figure in the field wrote, "The view now, within palliative medicine, is that it is okay to be symptomatologists—and proud of it." He continued, "Ultimately, suffering from losses, lack of love, existential doubts as well as from poverty and cruelty are not medical issues, and the response to them is not necessarily the responsibility of any healthcare discipline."[6] In the same vein, in discussing resource allocation and palliative care, others have ignored the spiritual domain and argued for a focus on symptom control, to the exclusion of even psychological concerns.[7]

The questions are basic. Does the spiritual/existential domain exist? Does it modify our experience of health, illness, suffering, and quality of life—including *all* symptoms, or doesn't it? Is the spiritual domain a determinant of the healing that can occur in dying? Are these issues essential to our understanding of health; to our understanding of health-care?

---

[2] Viktor Frankl, *The Doctor and the Soul*, 2nd expanded edition (Harmondsworth, UK: Pelican Books, 1973), p. 16.

[3] *Ibid.*, p. 9.

[4] World Health Organization, *Cancer Pain Relief and Palliative Care*, Technical Report Series 804 (1990), WHO, Geneva.

[5] Michael Kearney, "Palliative Medicine: Just Another Specialty?" *Palliative Medicine* 6(1) (1992): 39-46.

[6] Sam H. Ahmedzai, "Five Years: Five Threads", editorial, *Progress in Palliative Care*, 5(6) (1997): 235-237.

[7] C. Farsides and E. Garrard, "Resource Allocation in Palliative Care," in *New Themes in Palliative Care*, D. Clark, J. Hockley, S. Ahmedzai, eds. (Philadelphia: Open University Press, 1997), pp. 49-59.

In considering your response to these questions, let me introduce you to three people, each a person with cancer whom I have cared for, each my teacher about suffering and the potential we have to die healed.

I feel Chip's presence. I often do, although decades have passed since we last talked, just days before his death. "You know, Bal, this last year has been the best year of my life." Those last months had been agonizing for those of us who cared for Chip. We had been helpless as the apparent triumph of surgery and chemotherapy melted before our eyes. The physical magnificence of this gracious, world-class athlete and businessman had been reduced to a grotesque parody of his former impressive presence. The best year? Of that life? Chip explained that he had found himself on an unexpected journey inward. It was that voyage, he said, that had filled his dying with wonder and peace. He was thirty years old.

Then there was Anne. Seventy-two years old, this previously dynamic and independent woman was now trapped by metastatic breast cancer in a personal hell of bitterness, estrangement, and dependency. Month after month her dreadful quality of life haunted our attentive palliative care team. What more could we do? What were we missing? One of our senior nurses confided, "I don't believe in euthanasia, but Anne makes me wonder." Each carefully chronicled day seemed an eternity. Then, following months of anguish, within the space of twenty-four hours, there was a change. The nursing note read, "Better day today." Anne never looked back. Paradox! Each day, in the face of progressive physical weakness, her capacity to engage life grew. She worked with the art therapist, producing an impressive series of collages depicting life in all its fullness. The palliative care team was unable to account for her dramatic improvement. A detailed review of her care failed to reveal either a "breakthrough discussion" or a significant change in her physical status. The final weeks before her death were rich. Her daughter was overwhelmed with gratitude. "I can never thank you enough. You gave me the mother I never had. She has been a different person. We became friends. This was the most important experience of my life." What had turned the tragedy into success?

But all is not sweetness and light. I had been asked to see Mrs. L. by my palliative care colleague. Her pain was unrelieved in spite of the best efforts of a highly skilled team. It was due to cancer involving her bones and should have been easy to control. Why were we failing in this case? "When did you last feel well," I asked. She stiffened. Her eyes narrowed.

"Do you mean physically?" "That's an important question," I responded. "No, I mean in yourself." "Doctor," she cried, with obvious distress, "I have never been well a day in my life!" The depth of her anguish and the implications of her statement stunned me. "How distressing. If we are body, mind and spirit, where do you think the problem has been?" Without hesitation she shot back, "I have been sick in mind and spirit every day of my life!" I was moved. Impressed. What insight! Perhaps we could yet win this one. We never did control her pain. In spite of her insight, a life filled with disillusionment, anger, and defensive closing could not be mended at this late hour.

In 1996 Michael Kearney published *Mortally Wounded,* a landmark exploration of suffering and "soul pain" and the physician's role in their diagnosis and management.[8] In it he sounded a clarion call on behalf of a form of healthcare that fully considers body, mind, and spirit. He boldly asserted that it is *only* through attention to both the "surface" and the "deep" that sufferers can be enabled to become more fully themselves.

In *A Place of Healing* the memorable song of that first book becomes a full symphony. He accomplishes a breathtaking synthesis that draws on such wide-ranging fields as modern medicine, quantum physics, mythology, psychodynamic theory, and depth psychology as he further develops his vision of whole person care. In lucid prose Kearney lovingly builds his case, all the while taking care to trace the historical roots of this holistic approach back to the synthesis of Hippocratic medicine and Asklepian healing that lies at the germinal centre of his argument.

A Place of Healing brings us into the presence of the sacred. Are we human beings having spiritual experiences, or spiritual beings having human experiences? Either way, we can surely no longer ignore such questions. And, to quote J.W.N. Sullivan, "We can henceforth take but little account of attitudes toward life that leave no room for these experiences, attitudes which deny them or explain them away."[9]

This book deserves a wide readership. Michael Kearney is taking us to new depths, new heights. He takes us beyond the usual holistic care rhetoric. He takes us into uncharted territory and we find ourselves thankful for a guide who so uniquely combines breadth of vision, insight, sensitivity, and humility, as well as clarity of thought and expression.

---

[8] Michael Kearney, *Mortally Wounded: Stories of Soul Pain, Death and Healing* (Dublin: Marino Books, 1996).

[9] J.W.N. Sullivan, *Beethoven, His Spiritual Development* (New York: Random House, 1960), pp. 173-174.

Acknowledgments

I am indebted to many for help and inspiration with the original publication of this book. I especially want to thank my three beloved daughters, Mary-Anna, Claire, and Ruth, and their mother, Marian Dunlea, for their patience and support throughout. I am also very grateful to the following: Balfour Mount, Dympna Waldron, Maura McDonnell, Anne Hayes, Liam O' Siorain, Dierdre Horgan, Eithne Cunningham, Sr Francis Rose O' Flynn, the late Ursula Barry, Patrick Nolan, Patricia Skar, the late Sr Gabriel O' Mahony, Sr Mary Greaney, Helen Sands, Wendy Wilmott, and Marych O' Sullivan.

A special thank you to Nancy Cater for her generosity and support with this re-publication, and the many others whose behind the scenes efforts have made this a smooth and enjoyable process.

Finally, my heartfelt gratitude to Tom, Patricia, Rosalinda, Bill, and Mary, whose stories I share, with kind permission from their families, later in the book.

Illustrations

Page 33 Hippocrates: This statue was found on the island of Kos and is dated to the fourth century BC. It is exhibited in the Museum of Kos in the town of Kos. *Source:* C. Kerenyi (1959), *Asklepios: Archetypal Image of the Physician's Existence.* Copyright © 1959 by C. Kerenyi. Reprinted by Permission of Princeton University Press.

Page 40 Asklepios: This head of Asklepios was found on the island of Melos and is dated to approximately 340 B.C.E. It is exhibited at the British Museum in London. *Source:* Kerenyi (1959), p. 21.

Page 42 Asklepios with patient: A drawing from a votive relief now lost. From *Archiv fur Geschichte der Medizin, XVIII* (Leipzig, 1926). *Source:* Kerenyi (1959), p. 34.

Page 49 Intertwining Serpents: A wall plaque from the town of Kos, Island of Kos. Photographed by the author.

Page 55 Apollo: The Apollo Belvedere is dated to approximately 350 B.C.E. It is exhibited in the Vatican Museum in Rome. *Source:* Kerenyi (1959).

Page 56 Chiron: Painting from an Attic amphora and dated to approximately 520 B.C.E. From Furtängler and Reichhold, *Griechische Vasen-malerei,* text vol III (Munich, 1932). *Source:* Kerenyi (1959), p. 95.

Page 57 Hermes: A statue of a youthful Hermes. From the Vatican Museum in Rome. Photographed by the author.

Page 68 Dionysos: Painting from an Attic amphora by the Kleophrades painter dated to approximately 500 B.C.E. From the Glyptothek, Munich. *Source:* C. M. Bowra, *Classical Greece* (Amsterdam: Time-Life Books, 1965), p. 146. Staatliche Antiken sammlungen und Glyptothek Munchen.

Page 70 Demeter, Persephone and Triptolemus: The great Eleusinian relief, found at Eleusis and dated to approximately 440 B.C.E. It is exhibited at the National Archaeological Museum in Athens. Photographed by the author.

Page 74 Hygieia: A statue of Hygieia dated to approximately 250 C.E. It is exhibited at the Museum of Kos, in the town of Kos. Photographed by the author.

Page 77 Asklepios with serpent and staff: A statue of Asklepios from Epidauros and dated to the fourth century B.C.E. It is exhibited at the National Archaeological Museum in Athens. Photographed by Claire Kearney.

Page 90 Asklepios: Head of statue of Asklepios dated to approximately 250 B.C.E. It is exhibited at the National Archaeological Museum in Athens. Photographed by the author.

Page 269 Asklepian Temple: This is the remains of an Asklepian temple at Lissos, on the southwest coast of the Greek island of Crete. Photographed by the author.

Permissions

Introduction

I was twenty-three years old and coming to the end of my medical studies. I had become disillusioned with clinical medicine as I saw it practiced on the wards of the teaching hospitals and was considering leaving medical school to pursue my interests in English literature and film. An older man, whose advice I was seeking, suggested that before I do this, I should visit St. Christopher's Hospice in London, which he described as "a place of healing." I did as he suggested. While there I encountered patients who, despite the fact that their bodies were frail and dying, seemed to be among the most real and complete human beings I had ever met. I too felt more alive in their presence and left with my faith restored in the power of the human spirit—and in medical care. As I struggled afterwards to understand what had happened there, I found myself remembering my friend's words. A "place of healing" accurately described what I experienced during my visit, which had also rekindled an enthusiasm to continue with my medical training.

In many ways, that experience was the genesis of an exploration, both professional and personal, into the nature of healing and its place within healthcare. By "healing" here I mean the process of becoming psychologically and spiritually more integrated and whole; a phenomenon which enables persons to become more completely themselves and more fully alive. To speak of "healing in healthcare" may seem like a tautology. Surely, healing is what healthcare is all about? In my experience this is far from the truth. Western healthcare has become very focused on and very good at "curing," as in "fixing" and "making better," on restoring the sick person to the status quo of how life was before (or as close to this as possible). Contemporary western healthcare is not really that concerned with the question of healing. If healing happens in our healthcare institutions, it does so spontaneously and silently and is seen (if even recognized) as an idiosyncratic and unbidden bonus rather than a desired outcome.

A significant advance in healthcare in the latter part of the twentieth century has been the development of the hospice movement and the specialty of palliative care. From within this specialty a body of expertise has been established that can do much to control the pain and lessen the suffering of patients and families who are living with far advanced and terminal illness. For the past twenty years I have been working as a doctor in this area of care. On numerous occasions the experience of that early visit to St. Christopher's has been validated as I have witnessed patients becoming more human and alive, even as their bodies wasted away. This is not said to romanticize dying or in any way to minimize the distress of terminally ill patients and those close to them. Even for those patients receiving the "best possible" palliative care, some pain and suffering may remain, for ultimately dying is the greatest loss and the most absolute separation any of us can experience. What I am saying, however, is that even so, and even in the midst of such emotional distress and physical disintegration, even when nothing remains that can be "cured," "fixed," or "made better," this process of becoming more whole as human beings is witnessed by those caring for the dying again and again, and again.

I believe that palliative care is a microcosm of all healthcare where issues of broad relevance come into stark relief against a dark backdrop. Working with people approaching death, I have come to appreciate many of the strengths of the dominant paradigm of western healthcare, the so-called "medical model." These are evident in the multidisciplinary expertise that has been developed to treat and ease pain in its many forms. I have, however, also come to see the limitations of this model in this setting, particularly when confronted by certain forms of suffering, such as grief. Perhaps this is also true of the medical model in the broader context of general healthcare. While its strengths are again manifest in an ability to assess, explain, and successfully intervene in an ever-increasing range of problems, its limitations become apparent when confronted by forms of suffering that do not respond to such interventions. Failure to accept these limitations can lead to efforts that may prove counterproductive and damaging. On the other hand, an acceptance that the medical model, although valuable, is limited in what it can achieve in such circumstances, coupled with the observation that patients themselves often seem to find a way of living with and through their suffering to a place of greater wholeness, raises an important question. Is there another way, another model, besides the medical model, which is operative here and which could be of relevance when working with patients in intractable suffering?

Whether or not we even begin to search for such a model, however, is conditioned by how we view the responsibilities of healthcare. If we believe these are defined by that within the patient's experience of illness which responds to the interventions of the medical model—and it appears that many would accept such an analysis—then our task is relatively straight-forward. We must then use our considerable scientific and technological abilities to diagnose what can be diagnosed, cure what can be cured, fix what can be fixed and, when this is no longer possible, recognize that we have reached the limits of our abilities, do all we can to make the best of a difficult situation and hand over to others better qualified to deal with the patient's unresolved (and perhaps unresolvable) social, psychological, and existential issues. If you too share this viewpoint, perhaps you do not need to look beyond the medical model. If, however, you find such a position too narrow and believe that an attempt to work with the patient's *total* experience of illness, including those aspects of suffering that are unresponsive to the interventions of the medical model, *is* the concern of healthcare, then, I suggest, you must look for, identify, and learn to work with another model to partner the medical model. Were such a model to be found perhaps it could inform, deepen, and support a truly integrated clinical approach.

Where might we possibly begin our search for this other model? I suggest that we start in a place we may least expect to find it, that is, deep within the shadow cast by the luminous edifice of the medical model. If we look closely, we will discover there a narrow, winding pathway that leads us inwards, downwards, and backwards in time to ancient Greece and the very beginnings of western healthcare. There we find the two intertwined systems of early scientific or biomedical medicine, derived from the teachings of the great physician Hippocrates, and a form of psychological and spiritual healing based on the ritual practice of Asklepios, the Greek god of healing. Whereas Hippocratic medicine, representing the beginnings of the medical model, concentrated on the treatment of curable conditions, Asklepian healing was primarily concerned with helping those suffering from incurable conditions. Where Hippocratic practice emphasized the need for a rational and evidence-based approach and was dependent on an external agent to achieve its effect, the Asklepian rites assumed that there was a spontaneous tendency towards wholeness within each individual and that healing came through cooperation with this inner dynamic. Here was a culture that recognized the value of two fundamentally different but complementary models of care. Here was an integrated system of healthcare which attended to patients as whole persons: body, mind, soul, and spirit.

What of this ancient alliance and contemporary western healthcare? The reality is that these twin approaches which co-existed in a relationship of mutual respect and harmony in ancient Greece have, with the passing of time and as a result of a variety of historical developments, become widely split off and separated from each other. If the teaching of Hippocrates is clearly seen in the medical model, where, we may ask, are the healing rituals of Asklepios? At first glance it may appear as though Asklepios is long dead and buried and only remembered in the ruined healing temples of Greece. The presence of the god's emblem of the serpent coiled around a staff on the sides of our ambulances, the covers of our medical journals, and the windows of our pharmacies are, however, signs that this is not the case. Banished, perhaps, but not totally forgotten. Covertly, Asklepios is to be found within patients' subjective experiences of inner transformation and healing, and in the compassionate and caring attitude of those who attend them and stay with them in their suffering. Overtly, his influence is seen in areas such as the arts, the humanities, and deep ecology, as well as in body therapies, psychotherapies, and spiritual practice. Although many would consider these areas worthy and of value in themselves, few, I suspect, would view them as an essential and integral part of healthcare. I believe that for our system of western healthcare to truly become what its name implies we must consciously and deliberately begin to examine how we might welcome Asklepios back from the shadows. We would then have healthcare institutions that are not just places of caring, competence, and curing, but temples of healing also.

This book is written primarily for caregivers, whether professional or lay, who work with persons in suffering. It is also intended for those who are themselves living with suffering and for all who are interested in the inner quest for healing. The basic assumption underlying this way of working with suffering is that healing is something that happens, rather than something we do. Our role in this is to help create an environment where what is fundamental, natural, and indigenous to the human psyche can most easily do its own work of bringing about integration, balance, and wholeness.

Wherever a living creature—who might equally well be called a dying creature—is gravely ill, every turn for the better involves an element of mystery, even when the physician has recognized and eliminated the cause of the sickness. For the physician cannot act alone; side by side with his outside intervention something inside the patient must lend a helping hand if a cure is to be accomplished. At the crucial moment something is at work that might best be compared to the flow of a spring.

—CARL KERENYI, *Asklepios: Archetypal Image of the Physician's Existence*

SECTION I

CONTEXT

CHAPTER ONE

Beyond the Medical Model

I only want what is in your mind and in your heart.[1]

This was how a young Polish man dying with cancer replied to a question posed by his social worker. She had asked, "Is there anything else I can do to help you?" The patient's name was David Tasma and his social worker was Cicely Saunders. At this stage Saunders was planning to open a hospice where those with far-advanced and terminal illnesses could benefit from specialized treatments and multidisciplinary care. She had shared some of her plans with Tasma in the course of their many conversations. In one of their final encounters he had insisted that she accept £500, his life savings, as a donation to her new enterprise, adding, "I will be a window in your home."[2]

What are we to make of Tasma's cryptic words, which made such an impact on Saunders? She herself cites his request for knowledge combined with empathy as the inspiration for the system of "efficient loving care,"[3] which she went on to pioneer and tells of how his £500 did

---

[1] Shirley du Boulay, *Cicely Saunders* (London: Hodder and Stoughton, 1984), p. 56.
[2] *Ibid.*, p. 59.
[3] Cicely Saunders, *The Management of Terminal Malignant Disease*, 2nd ed. (London: Edward Arnold, 1984), p. 238.

indeed pay for a front window in St. Christopher's Hospice in London when it opened in 1967. I too hear in Tasma's words a request on behalf of all patients for a truly integrated approach to care. I also hear in what he says about being a window in the hospital, a metaphorical reminder of how patients *themselves* are an integral and essential part of the place and the process of healing.

THE MEDICAL MODEL AND THE PATIENT'S EXPERIENCE OF ILLNESS

As the dominant paradigm in western healthcare, the medical model reflects a wider value system, which prizes rational analysis and the ability to intervene in a logical way to change and control events. This is a highly successful paradigm, as is evident in its ability to prevent, treat, and cure an ever-expanding range of life-threatening illnesses and to significantly ease many previously uncontrolled forms of human misery. However, not all human distress is responsive to the interventions of the medical model, as is the case with certain forms of psychological and existential suffering. The strengths and limitations of the medical model in relation to the patient's experience of illness might, therefore, be represented diagrammatically in the following way:

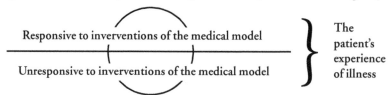

I would now like to introduce a possible shorthand way of talking about these two domains of a patient's experience of illness by considering the phenomena of pain and suffering.

Pain and Suffering

Pain as a physical symptom is defined by the International Association for the Study of Pain as:

> An unpleasant sensory and emotional experience associated with actual or potential *tissue damage*, or described in terms of such damage.[4]

---

[4] International Association for the Study of Pain Subcommittee on Taxonomy, "Pain terms: a list with definitions and notes on usage," *Pain* 8 (1980): 249-252.

According to this definition, pain is the experience that results from damage to a tissue, that is *part* of a person. When the damaged part is the liver we speak of "liver pain," when the damaged part is the bone we speak of "bone pain," and so forth. This definition also acknowledges that a crucial aspect of the experience of pain is in the person's sensory and emotional reaction to it. Saunders' use of the term *total pain*[5] further emphasizes how pain is a dynamic construct made up of interweaving layers of physical, social, emotional, and existential distress. The reality is that the vast majority of such pain can now be either fully controlled or at least very significantly eased using a multidisciplinary approach and the expertise accumulated in palliative care and specialist pain clinics.

- The first step in pain control is to fully *assess* the situation. Through careful listening to the patient's description, combined with clinical examination and, occasionally, some simple investigations, the underlying cause of the pain can be analyzed and its precise pathogenesis understood. For example, the *cause* of the pain may be correctly diagnosed as metastatic spread of cancer to the liver, but the *pathogenesis* of liver pain is stretching of the sensitive tissue, known as the visceral peritoneum, which encapsulates the liver.

- Having made this diagnosis, the next step is to *intervene* with appropriate treatment. "Appropriate" here refers both to the fact that the treatment should be a rational response to the underlying etiology of the pain and also that it should be proportionate to the overall clinical status of that individual patient.

- The third and final step is to regularly *reassess* and, if necessary, modify treatment in the light of the results achieved.

In summary, what we have seen is that pain affects *parts* of an individual. Using the principles of the medical model, pain can be assessed, treated, and in the vast majority of instances be brought under control. With pain, the answer lies outside the individual and is reliant primarily on the knowledge, skill, and intervention of another. The aim of such intervention is to alleviate the pain, thereby restoring that individual to a pain-free existence.

---

[5] Cicely Saunders, *The Management of Terminal Malignant Disease* (London: Edward Arnold, 1978), p. 194.

In contrast to pain, suffering can be understood as the experience that results from damage to the *whole* person. As physician Eric Cassell puts it, "Suffering occurs when the impending destruction of the person is perceived."[6] He continues, "Suffering can be defined as the state of severe distress associated with events which threaten the intactness of the person."[7]

Although there are aspects of suffering, which, like pain, can also be analyzed, understood and, through intervention, very significantly eased, many forms of suffering remain despite all efforts made by others and by individuals themselves. An example of this is grief. In the intense suffering of early grief an individual can feel as though his or her whole world has been torn apart. Pharmacological interventions do little to ease the intensity of this distress and make no impact whatsoever on the raw, open wound at the core of the experience.

We may speak of curing another's pain, but it is more appropriate to speak of individuals themselves finding healing within their suffering, for when healing comes to someone in suffering it does so from within the depths of his or her own psyche. This is not something that can be either predicted or prescribed. If it does occur, it happens spontaneously, in its own time and in its own way. To help someone in suffering, therefore, means creating the environment that best facilitates this process of inner healing. In practice this happens when a combination of effective care and human companionship helps to establish a secure, inner space for that person to be in. The process is further facilitated if the carers themselves have found ways of staying with and being in their own experience of suffering.

Diagrammatically, the relationship of pain and suffering to the medical model can be depicted in the following way:

Responsive to interventions of the medical model

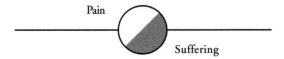

Unresponsive to interventions of the medical model

---

[6] Eric Cassell, *The Nature of Suffering and the Goals of Medicine* (Oxford, UK: Oxford University Press, 1991), p. 33.

[7] *Ibid.*

From what has been said here of pain and suffering, it is evident how, in addition to their literal meaning, these phenomena can be seen metaphorically. Throughout the remainder of this book, the term "pain" is used to describe both the symptom and/or those aspects of the patient's experience of illness that are responsive to the interventions of the medical model. Similarly, in addition to its literal meaning, the term "suffering" will be used to describe those aspects of the patient's experience of illness that are unresponsive to such interventions.

Tom's Story

The following case history illustrates the theoretical concepts discussed so far. As we consider how Tom lived with the pain and suffering engendered by far-advanced cancer, the strengths and limitations of the medical model become evident. We may also begin to discern the outlines of another model, which could inform our ways of working with suffering.

Tom in Pain

Tom was sixty-two years old. He was married to Claire and they had one son, John. Tom worked as a solicitor and possessed a precise and sharp intellect and a dry wit. He was a tall man, who had in his earlier years been a keen sportsman. He was obviously a quiet and private sort of person.

Three years previously a friend of Tom's had been diagnosed as having cancer of the prostate gland, on the basis of an elevated level of prostate specific antigen (the PSA level may be raised when there is cancer in the prostate gland). Shortly after this Tom had his PSA checked and was shocked and disappointed when this came back elevated. He was, however, reassured by his genito-urinary surgeon, who removed the tumor and told him that they had got the cancer at an early stage and that all should go well for him.

Sadly, this was not the case and approximately eighteen months later Tom developed backache. A bone scan showed secondary cancer in the vertebrae at the base of his spine and in his ribs, so his surgeon referred him to a radio-therapist who took over his care. Tom was treated with radiotherapy to his back and started on hormone therapy to try to prevent any further spread of the cancer. As his pain responded to this treatment, he was able to return to work.

Some months later, in October of that year, Tom's low back pain returned but this time was very much more severe. As well as arranging for Tom to have a further course of radiotherapy, his family doctor organized for the home care team from the local palliative care unit to visit and advise on his pain control. On their advice, he was commenced on regular morphine, in conjunction with the anti-inflammatory drugs he was already taking. Since his pain did not respond to this intervention, a respite admission to the palliative care unit for assessment and symptom control was organized.

During this admission, the staff found Tom somewhat anxious and slow to trust them. He was, understandably, very focused on his pain and impatient with the lack of success of various changes of his medications. Ultimately what made the difference was treatment with intravenous strontium, a radioactive isotope, which was organized and given by Tom's radiotherapist during an outpatient visit to the nearby radiotherapy unit. He returned home shortly after this, his pain much reduced, and was able to recommence work soon afterwards.

Three months later, in February of the following year, Tom was readmitted to the palliative care unit because of a return of incapacitating low back pain, now radiating down both his legs. He was very frightened by the pain, which was there constantly as a low-grade constant ache but which broke through occasionally with severe exacerbations. Radiographs did not show any evidence of spinal collapse. Both Tom and Claire were anxious for him to have another strontium treatment, because this had previously been so successful, and the radiotherapist was consulted. He did not feel that he could repeat this since Tom's bone marrow was showing signs of reduced activity, perhaps as a consequence of the previous treatment. He did, however, give Tom a further small dose of radiotherapy to his spine, hoping this would make a difference. He also warned that any further treatment to that part of his spine ran the risk of damaging the spinal cord.

Meanwhile in the palliative care unit we were adjusting Tom's medications to try and achieve maximum benefit with a minimum of side-effects. On the higher doses of morphine he had become drowsy and he disliked this intensely. We changed him to an alternative strong opioid, which he tolerated better and gave a treatment with intravenous bisphosphonates, drugs which can help pain due to bone destruction. With all these interventions Tom's pain lessened and he began to mobilize. Frail but more comfortable, he was discharged home after just less than two weeks in the unit. He was still hopeful that he would continue to improve to the point of returning to work at some future date.

Sadly, within forty-eight hours, Tom had to be readmitted as an emergency to the palliative care unit. His pain had worsened in intensity to the point that he was now terrified to move. As well as constant severe low back pain, he was also having intermittent piercing jabs of pain, which spread down his buttocks and into the backs of both his legs. An anesthetist, who was also a pain specialist, was asked to review Tom and he inserted an epidural catheter, a little plastic tube placed beneath the skin to lie close to the spinal cord, at the approximate level of origin of the pain. The constant infusion of morphine and local anesthetic through this gave good pain relief. However, by then a new problem was developing. Tom began to complain that his legs felt weak. He was examined carefully by the doctor on call who did not find any objective leg weakness. These findings, coupled with the fact that Tom was able to walk, with assistance, to the bathroom led to the conclusion that the subjective sensation of weakness was most likely due to the local anesthetic infusion and so, on consultation with the anesthetist, this was withdrawn from the epidural pump.

The following morning, Tom awoke to find that he could barely move his legs. He was immediately started on high dose corticosteroids, on the assumption that this might indicate pressure on his spinal cord and an emergency magnetic resonance imaging (MRI) scan was organized. He had the scan early that afternoon and it showed a tumor growing from the vertebrae at the base of his spine, encircling his spinal cord at that level. Immediately after this, Tom was seen by his radiotherapist who, on the basis of the precise location of the spinal involvement on the scan, was able to give some further radiotherapy. He had his first of five radiotherapy treatments at this stage and then returned to the palliative care unit.

I recall sitting with Tom and Claire later that evening. It was as though the previous days, indeed weeks, had been a helter-skelter of activity as Tom had been hurled by his illness from one crisis to the next. Suddenly there was a pause in this chaotic spiral of out-of-control events, and silence. I recall Tom, eyes slightly widened as if in shock, turning in slow motion towards me and asking "What now?" I suspected the worst; that this was a catastrophic development and that there was little hope of recovery and every possibility that things could only further deteriorate. I could not bring myself to say this to Tom, and, indeed, it would have been entirely inappropriate to do so. I responded at a practical level, describing again what was going on and how we all hoped the combination of steroids and radiotherapy would relieve the pressure on his spinal cord and so allow the nerves to his legs to regain some of their function. Disbelief, numbness, horror were what I saw on Tom's face as he turned away from me to look at Claire. She was leaning forward at the other side of his bed, holding his hand and with a calm strength reinforcing the positive aspects of what I had just said and somehow even managing to bring in a flash of humour and a brief smile to Tom's lips.

Towards the end of the week I called in to see Tom late in the afternoon. By then he had almost completed his radiotherapy treatments but with no benefit. What little bit of power he had that previous Monday morning had gone and with it all sensation from his waist down. No longer having any rectal sensation, he had been incontinent of feces without even being aware of it. At least a urinary catheter had given him some control of his bladder function. Ironically, the only benefit of his new situation was that because of the numbness he was now completely free of physical pain.

Although the physical numbness from his waist down was by then complete, it appeared that the emotional numbness engendered by recent events was wearing off. Tom was devastated. It was as though he was now seeing within and beyond the awful reality of what had happened a black abyss that had opened up beneath him. Turning slowly to look down at the shape of his legs under the sheets in front of him, he said: "It is as though I am dead from the waist down. I am looking down on my dead lower half. This is worse than anything I could have possibly imagined. I was ready to die, but not—ever—*this*. I can't go on like this. I want to walk again or to die. I can't go on like this."

Listening to Tom I too felt numb and impotent. I could say or do nothing except agree with him that it was horrible, the most awful thing that could have happened. I sat with him a while, both of us now silent. Reassuring him that I would call back the following morning, I left him alone.

The effectiveness of the medical model is apparent in the early diagnosis and treatment of Tom's cancer. It is what subsequently facilitated the prompt diagnosis and treatment of the cancer recurrence. Finally, even in the very advanced stages of the disease, it is what enabled the accurate assessment of the spinal cord compression and attempts at palliation. Although Tom's goals may have changed from curing the cancer, to treating the secondaries, to controlling the pain, to walking again, he was consistent in his expectation, throughout the trajectory of his illness, that the medical model would restore, in some shape and form, the life he had known before. Up to this point, the medical model had served Tom well. It had allowed him to live a relatively normal life during most of the three years of his incurable illness and even in the later stages of the illness it had continued to bring him some relief and comfort.

Tom in Suffering

I called back to see Tom the next day and on each of the days that followed. On every occasion we would begin by talking about what was happening in a practical, material sense. By now it was clear to all that there would be no improvement in his paraplegia. Each new day confronted him with further implications of his utter dependency on others. For example, he now needed to be transferred by the nurses using a mechanical hoist to the commode or to sit out in a chair next to his bed. His sadness and the sense of the unfairness and utter meaninglessness of what had happened were by now tangible. His worst fear of the future was that it would continue like this. There was nothing I could say to comfort him. Even attempts to reassure him about these fears by saying that "it wouldn't go on all that long" backfired when he pressed me to clarify what I meant by this and I answered "weeks rather than months." It was evident from his groan-like response that this sounded like an eternity, and hell. By going over the same ground, by asking the same questions again and again, Tom was struggling to make some sense of what was happening, to find some scrap of consolation or comfort in his suffering. His questions to me at this stage were clearly rhetorical. He had already discovered that I did not have the answers.

A few days later Tom turned to me and asked, "And what's going to happen next?" He had asked me this before and I had answered him in practical and objective terms. This time I decided to take a risk and replied that we could look at the time ahead in two ways: in terms of "outer work" and in terms of "inner work". The outer work was a continuation of what he was already doing as he worked with the nursing staff and the physiotherapist to find the easiest and best ways of living with his disability and of maximizing what power and ability he still had. The inner work was about trying to find some way through his feelings of grief, disappointment, and black despair. I told him of patients I had cared for who *had* come through and that although it might seem impossible to even imagine such an outcome, it had happened for others before him. I attempted to explain this in the following way:

> Whatever it is that helps people through this blackness to a place where they can live more easily, even at peace with how it is, seems to come from deep within individuals themselves. It is as though there is some inner strength or wisdom which is particularly available in times of crisis like this, some inner understanding that wants to help us, if we can only allow it. For our part, all that is possible is to do the outer work to the best of our ability while beginning to find ways of co-operating with this inner work. This is a bit like starting to learn a new language, or trying to see in the dark or tuning in a radio to a new station—one that we hadn't even known existed.

I reassured Tom at this point that this inner work would happen *anyway* and that this seemed to be something that occurred imperceptibly and naturally within us. I used the example of a seed that has germinated in the darkness of the earth and is already pushing its way with its own energy towards the surface. I added: "Perhaps our efforts don't so much affect whether or not this will happen, as how and when it will happen."

It was evident that Tom was interested in what I was saying and he asked me what "tuning in to this wavelength" meant in practical terms. I suggested that he might begin to keep a journal of what seemed like significant thoughts, feelings, or memories that occurred to him during the day, and in particular that he make a note of any dreams he remembered, either first thing in the morning or after sleeping during the day. In addition, I suggested that he might like to meet the art therapist, adding that there were many different ways of "tuning in" and that it was really about experimenting until he found a way that he was comfortable with. I remember how he looked at me at this point, his head tilted a little back and to one side and with a slight smile, which could have meant many things; perhaps humorous disbelief or maybe the shyness of one who is about to embark on something, which, despite the learned doctor's explanations, seemed utterly *ridiculous!*

We had this conversation about "inner work" on a Wednesday afternoon. I mentioned to him that I would be away from the end of that week for a fortnight but arranged that we would meet for an hour before I left to discuss how he was getting on.

As I entered his room that Friday morning, Tom leant over towards his bedside locker and picked up a copybook and waved it in the air towards me. "My journal!" he declared, adding somewhat triumphantly that he had not had a single dream since he got it. He mentioned that the last dreams he could remember were from about two weeks previously, around the time he had lost the use of his legs. I asked him to describe what he could remember of these dreams. He began:

> They don't mean anything … In the first of these I'm in the house I grew up in (until I was about seventeen years old). It was a big, old rambling country house. There were always jobs and repairs to be done. I was the eldest—I had a younger brother and two sisters. What surprised me was that, when I awoke, I could remember this house so vividly, whereas I couldn't visualize my present house and I really felt I needed to. There are so many practical things to be considered, such as, will my wheelchair fit through the front door? The harder I tried to visualize my present house, the less I was able and that made me feel frustrated, panicky … helpless. I was utterly powerless. Then I went back to sleep. I was in and out of these thoughts and feelings all night long. It even lasted into the following day … I was haunted by it …
>
> The other one was vague. I only remember impressions. To talk about it, even that seems too specific. I was standing beside a mound of leftover tarmac. There were three holes in it. That detail seemed definite and felt important. There were also three poplar trees growing out of it. I was drawn to look upwards with them. Claire is there with some of her friends—possibly bridge-friends— and they seem to be managing, to be getting somewhere. I'm there with some of my friends but it's like we're stuck; we're getting nowhere. I feel frustrated, useless …

As I listened it occurred to me that the feelings Tom described in his dreams were similar to the feelings I had felt as I had sat with him in the immediate aftermath of his paralysis. As he finished, he turned and looked in my direction. His eyebrows were raised expectantly as though waiting for me to offer some sort of interpretation.

> The dream itself is what matters here, Tom. It's not about me
> offering my interpretation. What's important, as psychologist James
> Hillman says, is "keeping the dream alive."[8] If dreams really are
> messages from our deeper selves, then it's as though the images in
> the dreams themselves embody this message. What we need to do,
> as you are doing, is to give them attention by remembering the
> images and by noticing the feelings that come with them. This seems
> to be what "tuning in" means here.

In view of my imminent departure, I was keen to show Tom a
simple method of dreamwork in practice so that he could, if he so chose,
reflect on his dreams in this way in my absence. I asked him which
dream image he would like to look at. He said he would like to look
at the dream of the tarmac. I asked him to describe anything in the
dream that seemed important to him, in as much detail as he could
and to notice if he felt anything in particular as he did so. He spoke of
the three holes in the tarmac; they *felt* really important, but he couldn't
say why. *The three poplars; these were huge trees, tall, upright;* he spoke
of how they had recently had three poplars cut down from outside
the front of their house; they had got so big, they were blocking the
light. *Claire and her bridge friends and he and his friends;* his feelings of
getting nowhere, of uselessness, of frustration: these images, he said,
didn't seem to make any sense at all. At this point I asked him if he
saw or perhaps felt any connections between the images and feelings
in the dream and his situation around the time he had the dream, or
indeed since. He replied that he could not see any such connections
and then began talking about his first meeting with the art therapist
the day previously: "I found it disturbing. Why do I need to stir up
my emotions when they are already so raw?"

I felt that Tom was also saying something to me in this, that
perhaps my question about the feelings in the dream and his present
situation might have been too confronting. Maybe, in my anxiety
about leaving him at this stage, I was pushing the pace too quickly for
him. I reassured him that the inner work was happening anyway and
that whatever else he did to co-operate with this had to feel safe to
him. He said he had decided to give the art therapy a break for the
time being. Meanwhile he would see what happened with his dreams.

---

[8] James Hillman, *The Dream and the Underworld* (New York: Harper and Row,
1979), p. 116.

On returning to work two weeks later, I telephoned ahead to the ward to see how Tom was. He had just died. I went to the ward and heard from Maura, the ward sister, how the last two weeks had been. Apparently he had remained very comfortable during this time, with no further pain. He seemed to have come to a place of peace in himself and was very open to the nurses and their care. Maura's feeling was that his openness to being cared for physically marked a change in Tom. She felt he had "mellowed" and become more receptive. Two days previously Tom had commented wryly to Maura that "This spectacle is more difficult for the onlookers than it is for the patient." Hours later he had started to bleed from his bowel. He had been so weak at this stage that he was unaware of what was happening. The decision not to treat this with blood transfusions had been agreed with Claire. She and John had been with him throughout the last few days and were with him when he died.

I went to the ward and called into Tom's room. He was lying, as if asleep with his son sitting close by. As I stood there, John commented that the paraplegia was the worst thing that could have happened to his father, "Up until then he always thought he was going to get over it." Tom's hand was still warm as I touched him and said a silent goodbye. When I left the room I met Claire in the corridor. She thanked us for all we had done and said:

> A few days ago I was sitting with Tom. He seemed so serene and I asked him "Are you in pain?"
>
> "No" he replied.
>
> "Are you at peace?"
>
> "Yes, he replied.
>
> "Are you happy?"
>
> "No," he said.
>
> "And I'm afraid he had not written a single word in his journal," Claire added finally and almost apologetically.

She turned and went back into Tom's room.

Although the medical model helped significantly in the earlier phase of Tom's illness and in a variety of ways throughout the later and terminal stages, its limitations became evident in the face of the insoluble problems of his spinal cord compression and the resulting emotional and psychological torment. At this stage it became increasingly clear that there simply were no answers to so many of his questions, and that any further interventions would be futile. All that the carers could now do was to continue to treat what problems could be treated, and to stay with Tom in his suffering.

Then something very curious began to happen. In the days that followed, Tom seemed to move gradually, and almost imperceptibly, through his struggle and distress to an easier place within himself; a place of peace and sadness. What had happened here? What had made the difference? Was it something "mysterious" that defies description or are there elements of this process which can be identified? Attempting to understand what happened for Tom, as with many such similar situations encountered in clinical practice, may help us to see what can facilitate such a process.

Firstly, there was Tom's remarkable personal courage (which at times meant being afraid, frustrated, and hopeless—and feeling it) and the constant, loving support of his family. There was the secure environment created by the medical model through effective, multidisciplinary palliative care. There was an appreciation by the caring team of the limits of the medical model in the face of suffering, coupled with an intuitive faith on their part, and based on previous clinical and perhaps personal experience, that there was "another way". There was a sense that this included a continuing to care and to do all that was possible to minimize distress; a valuing of human relationship, of presence and of caring physical contact and an ability to acknowledge as carers the painful feelings of impotence and outrage in witnessing another's suffering without having to act on them. There was also a trusting that time and something *within Tom himself* could, and might, bring about change.

With David Tasma, Tom wanted of his carers help in his *total* experience of illness; that is, in both his pain *and* his suffering. Although we have come a long way in our ability to describe, analyze, and treat pain, we still find ourselves hesitant and inarticulate when we begin to address the question of suffering. Nonetheless, I agree with Eric Cassell who puts it starkly:

> The test of a system of medicine should be its adequacy in the face
> of suffering; ... modern medicine fails that test. In fact, the central

assumptions on which twentieth-century medicine is founded
provide no basis for an understanding of suffering. For pain, difficulty
in breathing, or other afflictions of the body, superbly *yes;* for
suffering, no.[9]

If we are to find creative and effective ways of working with patients
in suffering, we must describe more accurately and understand in
greater depth the "other way, the "second model," which became
operative alongside the medical model during Tom's final weeks. In the
following chapter, I shall consider some possible ways of doing this.

---

[9] Eric Cassell, p. vii.

CHAPTER TWO

Ways of Seeing

We might say that at this moment, as in the time of Galileo, what we most urgently need is much less new facts (there are enough and even embarrassingly more than enough of these in every quarter) than a new way of looking at the facts and accepting them. *A new way of seeing, combined with a new way of acting—that is what we need.*

—Teilhard de Chardin[1]

People in pain and suffering need both what the medical model and this other, at present unnamed model of healing have to offer. This means effective pain control and an approach that lessens the suffering and helps that individual to endure, live with and hopefully, in time, live through that suffering. To fully realize the potential of such an integrated approach in healthcare, we need to find accurate ways of describing these two contrasting paradigms of care. How we see something and how we name and speak of that thing matters. The language we use reveals our attitude. This influences how we, and in turn others, see, value, and respond to this particular thing. We can speak of these twin models of care in a variety of ways. Each of these can complement the other and help paint a more complete picture of what it is we are trying to describe.

---

[1] Pierre Teilhard de Chardin, *Activation of Energy* (London: Collins, 1970), pp. 294-295.

A Psychological Metaphor

There a number of possible ways of examining the two paradigms of healthcare through psychological concepts. We could compare the medical model to normal ego-functioning within the conscious mind and the healing model to the more mysterious workings of the unconscious. Alternatively, we could draw comparisons between the medical model and the left-brain functions of logical and analytical thinking and the healing model and the intuitive, symbolic, and lateral-thinking functioning of the right brain. Another way of speaking of these two models is to consider the human psyche in terms of its *surface* and *depth* dimensions. This can be illustrated diagrammatically in the following way:

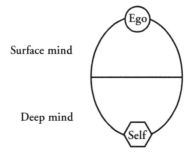

Here the term *surface mind* describes the rational and literal aspects of the mind. The strengths of the surface mind are in its ability to analyze and understand. Communication within and from the surface mind is through words, which express logical concepts. This is the dimension of mind that is operative in normal waking consciousness. The *ego* is the aware and discriminating part of the mind. It is at home in the surface mind, which is familiar territory and where things *usually* work in predictable and orderly ways. The ego feels in control in the surface mind.

The term *deep mind* describes the normally unconscious and intuitive aspects of the mind. It is intimately connected to the emotions and the physical body. Its operative vocabulary is image, symbol, and myth. This is the dimension of mind that is active in nocturnal dreaming and waking fantasy and imaginative and creative activities. Within the deep mind resides what the pioneering depth psychologist Carl Jung called the *Self.* Jungian analyst Jane Hollister Wheelwright speaks of the Self as the:

> [A]rchetype of wholeness and order, at once the centre and container of the totality of the psyche. The [S]elf is a function, uniting all pairs of opposites, of a source of energy, which is the instigator and director of the individuation process. It is manifested by way of projection, by means of symbols ... and by the conflict of opposites ... Jung has referred to the [S]elf as "the God within us."[2]

The comparison between the ego and the surface mind with the workings of the medical model is evident. Perhaps we could also compare the healing model to the workings of the deep mind and the Self. What we then have are two very different systems working side by side; one with the ability to analyze, separate, and cure, another with the ability to understand, include, integrate, and heal.

Further consideration of this psychological metaphor, however, reveals a possible explanation why, in reality, the medical model is the only recognized model within western healthcare. For not only is the ego at home and in control in the surface mind, it is also terrified of the deep mind. The ego sees the deep mind as a dark, fathomless abyss and a dustbin of psychic waste and nightmares. In a situation of illness, and especially in the crisis of a life-threatening illness, the ego can project its fear of the unknown on to the deep mind in a well-described psychological defense mechanism known as "terror management."

Terror Management Theory

Three sociologists, Solomon, Greenberg and Pyszczynski, have built on the pioneering work of Ernest Becker[3] to develop what they call *terror management theory.*[4] In this they postulate that a defining characteristic of human beings is a capacity for "mortality salience," that is, the ability to be aware of one's own mortality. This awareness generates "terror," which they describe not as an intense fear of death, *per se,* but rather as a profound and usually unconscious dread of death as absolute annihilation. We cope, they suggest, with such terror by developing what they term an "anxiety buffer." This is achieved by

[2] Jane Hollister Wheelwright, *The Death of a Woman* (New York: St. Martin's Press, 1981), pp. 284-285.

[3] Ernest Becker, *The Denial of Death* (New York: Free Press Paperbacks, 1973).

[4] S. Solomon, J. Greenberg, and T. Pyszczynski, "Terror management theory of self-esteem," in *Handbook of Social and Clinical Psychology: The Health Perspective*, ed. C. R. Synder and D. Forsyth (New York: Pergamon, 1991), pp. 21-40.

denying or repressing the terror at an individual level while simultaneously creating, maintaining, and participating in "culture" at a communal level. From their perspective, culture is seen as a symbolic perceptual construct, the primary purpose of which is to minimize the anxiety associated with an awareness of death. This it does by bestowing on the individual within that culture a sense of "self-esteem." By having faith in the cultural world view and accepting the standards of value inherent in that world view, the individual is rewarded by gaining a sense of meaning; perceiving that one is meeting those standards and therefore playing a significant role in the cultural conception of reality also brings with it a sense of personal value. Self-esteem, therefore, arises from viewing oneself as a valued participant in a meaningful cultural drama. This minimizes death anxiety by giving us a sense of safety and of being part of something greater that will not die; that is, a reassurance of immortality. It follows from this that one of the primary motivations of human behaviour is to defend the death anxiety buffer by maintaining self-esteem.

Solomon and his colleagues have shown that threats to self-esteem heighten an individual's anxiety, which in turn activates defenses (what they call "terror management processes"). These work to minimize the anxiety by restoring the status quo. In addition, in a fascinating series of studies, they have shown that when individuals become mortality salient, that is when the individuals' denial is threatened by reminding them of their mortality, these same terror management processes are also triggered. These defense or terror management processes have consistently been shown to maintain self-esteem, and so lessen anxiety, in two principal ways:

- by reinforcing the dominant cultural world views
- by distancing oneself from or denigrating alternative views.

To illustrate how terror management processes work, Solomon and his colleagues tell of a study performed with a group of North American municipal court judges. One group of judges had been made mortality salient, the other group had not. Both groups were then asked to recommend a dollar amount at which bail should be set for a woman accused of prostitution. The study showed that the mortality salient group of judges was significantly more punitive to the woman accused of prostitution (i.e., someone whom they saw as threatening cultural norms and therefore self-esteem). These findings were later replicated in studies with mortality salient college students, who were also significantly more positive than the control group in rewarding an individual who had heroically attempted to uphold cultural values.[5]

What is the relevance of this to the psychological metaphor of the surface and deep aspects of mind? Terror management theory demonstrates how efforts are made by mortality salient individuals to lessen death-induced anxiety by punishing those who threaten and rewarding those that uphold their cultural norms, thereby bolstering their protective self-esteem buffer. In terms of the western psyche, the dominant cultural values are those of the surface mind; that is of rational, analytic, linear, and concrete thinking. The reaction of the ego when it senses death's approach (i.e., becomes mortality salient) bears a striking resemblance to that of a mortality salient municipal judge in the studies by Solomon and his colleagues. At an intrapsychic level, this is seen in the mortality salient ego's clinging to the values of the surface mind while simultaneously projecting onto the deep mind the face of a terrifying enemy, rejecting its values, and distancing itself from what it sees as a threatening and potentially destructive aspect of psyche. In other words, in a frantic attempt to lessen anxiety, the ego projects its fear of death on to the deep and unconscious aspects of mind, seeing in its unfamiliar and unpredictable depths a microcosm of death itself. In this reaction aimed at ensuring its survival, the panicking ego flees from the deeper layers of the psyche, thereby alienating itself from a potential source of profound inner healing, which contact with this aspect of the psyche can bring.

The possibility that terror management processes are also active in individuals working within western healthcare would help to explain the dehumanizing excesses of technological medicine as the defensive activities of terrified human egos made mortality salient by constant proximity to disease and death. It also explains the complete dominance of the medical model within healthcare, as this closely reflects the prevailing culture of the surface mind. This might also help us to

---

[5] S. Solomon, J. Greenberg, and T. Pyszczynski, "A terror management theory of social behaviour: the psychological functions of self-esteem and cultural worldviews," in *Advances in Experimental Social Psychology,* ed. M. P. Zanna (San Diego: Academic Press, 1991), p. 127.

understand why a splitting occurs between the medical model and systems of care and therapeutic approaches which embody the values of the minority culture, the deep mind. At best these approaches are denigrated as "soft" (i.e., tolerated within the system but, by implication, not really that important or relevant in the real world of "hard data"); at worst they are rubbished as "useless" or even "dangerous."

A SCIENTIFIC METAPHOR

Another useful way of looking at and speaking of the two models of healthcare is from within a scientific framework. Here we see parallels between the medical model and classical physics and can learn more of the healing model by considering some of the insights of the new physics.

Classical Physics

> The strongest influences in our modern culture derive from the philosophical and scientific revolution of the seventeenth century, from the cultivation of Cartesian doubt and the birth of Newtonian, or classical, physics.
>
> —DANAH ZOHAR[6]

In 1687 Isaac Newton published a work entitled *Principia* in which he outlined his three laws of motion. These were:

1. *The law of inertia.* If undisturbed, a material body will continue to move in a straight line at constant speed.
2. *The law of acceleration.* Alterations in speed and direction are caused by and proportional to applied forces. Acceleration is inversely proportional to mass, i.e., it is more difficult to change the course of a heavy moving body than a light one.
3. *The law of action and reaction.* For every action there is an equal and opposite reaction (e.g., if I push something, it pushes back equally on me).[7]

With these three laws, and building on the work of others including Copernicus and Galileo, Newton heralded a world view that has dominated western thinking for the past 300 years and the

---

[6] Danah Zohar, *The Quantum Self* (London: Flamingo, 1991), p. 1.

[7] Ian Marshall and Danah Zohar, *Who's Afraid of Schrödinger's Cat?* (London: Bloomsbury, 1997), p. 11.

ramifications of which have been felt in every sphere of life. The "Newtonian" or "classical" view can be summarized as seeing the universe as:

> So many isolated and impenetrable atoms that bounce around in space and collide with one another like tiny billiard balls. The *only* actors in Newton's space-time drama were such particles and the attractive or repulsive forces acting between them.[8]

Newton's world was understood on the basis of observation and analysis of concrete data:

> [It] was thought to consist of many observable data that could be analyzed and reduced to a few simple laws and principles, or to a few basic components. The laws and principles became the basis for all-embracing general theories and sets of predictions that could be tested through experiments, which were conducted strictly in accordance with a new scientific method that viewed systems in isolation from their environments, breaking them down into their simplest component parts and using the behaviour of these parts to predict the unfolding future of the system.
>
> Simplicity, determinism, and predictability were the cornerstones of the Newtonian approach. Any system or object starting from some given state or position and acted upon by some given force would always behave in exactly the same way. Cause and effect reigned supreme, and there was always a direct, linear relationship between the force acting upon a body (the cause) and the deflection of that body from its original course (the effect).[9]

We can recognize the mechanistic paradigm of Newtonian physics dealing with space and time, solid matter, and cause and effect, as the same paradigm that informs the medical model. Newton's careful observations of the properties of matter and his declaration that such empirical data was what must form the basis of our knowledge and action in the world, is one and the same as that of contemporary, biomedical, evidence-based medicine.

The New Physics

The "new" physics is in fact about 100 years old. It represents a second scientific revolution and introduces a new paradigm that is

---

[8] Danah Zohar and Ian Marshall, *The Quantum Society* (London: Flamingo, 1994), p. 4.
[9] Ian Marshall and Danah Zohar, pp. xix-xx.

radically different from that of classical physics. Although many of the central concepts of the new physics seem to "make sense" at first glance, they are often difficult to understand and may, on reflection, seem illogical and confusing. This certainly has been my own experience. For me, reading the new physics has been similar to reading poetry. In my heart I respond enthusiastically to what is being revealed, but my head becomes progressively more perplexed as it struggles, unsuccessfully, to fit the data into rational and logical concepts. I have found the writings of philosopher and physicist Danah Zohar and psychiatrist and mathematician Ian Marshall enormously helpful here. They emphasize that to approach the new physics we need a different mode of understanding, what is called "fuzzy logic":

> Quantum mechanics is counterintuitive, or a strain on common sense ... In ordinary experience, things behave like waves *or* particles. ... Ordinary logic, like our everyday experience ... is an either/or logic ... But there is a newer branch of logic, known as fuzzy logic, that deals with superpositions and matters of degree. This is a both/ and or wave like logic.[10]

> Like Buddhism and Eastern mysticism in general, fuzzy logic is at home with contradictions. It is a logic that stresses matters of degree and all those shades of grey in between black and white.[11]

The term "new physics" refers both to Einstein's relativity theory and to quantum mechanics. What primarily concerns us here is the latter, i.e., the world of quantum mechanics that describes "The physics of the micro-world within the atom, that is the inner workings of everything we see and, at least physically, are."[12]

Whereas Newtonian physics saw atoms as the billiard balls and building blocks of physical reality which operated in linear and predictable ways, the behaviour of atoms in quantum physics is very different. The most essential differences are seen in examining a number of key concepts, as outlined by Zohar and Marshall.

---

[10] *Ibid.*, p. 339.
[11] *Ibid.*, p. 162.
[12] Zohar, p. 4.

Waves and Particles

> All being at the subatomic level can be described equally well either
> as solid particles, like so many minute billiard balls, or as waves,
> like undulations on the surface of the sea.[13]

Waves and particles are not the invention of quantum physics. Both exist in the Newtonian physics but the very different way in which they are viewed highlights the contrasting perspectives of both paradigms. In Newton's physics, particles are the most fundamental building blocks of matter and their interactions occur along the predictable lines of the three laws of motion, as already discussed. Waves, on the other hand, such as light waves, are "thought to be vibrations in some underlying "jelly" (the ether), not fundamental things in themselves."[14] Thus, from the Newtonian perspective, matter and light are *either* particle *or* wave and while both waves and particles have a role to play in Newtonian physics, particles are thought to be the more basic.

Although there is no dispute that light and matter are composed of both waves and particles, their function and fundamental status are viewed quite differently in quantum physics. The "particle" aspect of an object is its static, concrete, actual presence in the here and now of space and time; the "wave" aspect of the same object is its dynamic, fluid nature existing, simultaneously, in equally real, but very different realms of space and time. Furthermore:

> Quantum physics goes on to tell us that neither description is really
> accurate on its own, that both the wave-like and the particle-like
> aspects of being must be considered when trying to understand the
> nature of things, and that it is the duality itself which is the most
> basic. Quantum "stuff" is, essentially, *both* wave-like and particle-
> like, simultaneously.[15]

This concept is one of quantum physics' most revolutionary ideas and is called the "wave/particle duality":

> All the constituents of matter and light are *both* wave-like *and*
> particle-like *at the same time*. … Neither aspect of the duality—the
> wavelike or the particle-like—is more primary or more real. The

---

[13] *Ibid.*, p. 9.
[14] *Ibid.*, p. 10.
[15] *Ibid.*, p. 9.

two complement each other, and both are necessary for any full
description of what light and matter really are.[16]

When two objects meet, they do so in both aspects of their nature.
Since particles are localized to one point in space and time when they
meet, they:

> bump into each other, clash, and go their separate ways. Waves
> [however] are not localized; they can spread out across vast regions
> of space and time. When two meet, they can overlap and pass
> through each other. ... Particles are always individuals, but since
> any two wave patterns add up to make a third, waves are not.[17]

Particles are therefore discrete and separate, but waves connect and merge.
In quantum terminology this phenomenon is called "relational holism":

> Every quantum entity has both a wavelike and a particle-like aspect.
> The wavelike aspect is indeterminate, spread out all over space and
> time and the realm of possibility. The particle-like aspect is
> determinate, located at one place in space and time and limited to
> the domain of actuality. The particle-like aspect is fixed, but the
> wavelike aspect becomes fixed only in dialogue with its
> surroundings—in dialogue with an experimental context or in
> relationship to another entity in measurement or observation. It is
> the indeterminate, wavelike aspect—the set of potentialities
> associated with the entity—that unites quantum things or systems
> in a truly emergent, relational holism that cannot be reduced to
> any previously existing parts or their properties.[18]

> The whole of quantum reality is to some extent an unbroken web
> of overlapping or correlated, internal relationship. It has what David
> Bohm calls a quality of "undivided wholeness."[19]

The Quantum Vacuum and Quantum Field Theory

Although particles and waves fill the universe with all we see and
know, at the core of the quantum universe there is an empty space, a
no-thingness that is full of all possibility. Zohar and Marshall describe
this as:

> The ground state of energy in the universe, the lowest possible level,
> [and it] is known as the quantum vacuum. It is called a vacuum

---

[16] Marshall and Zohar, p. 384.
[17] *Ibid.*, p. 385.
[18] *Ibid.*, p. 186.
[19] Zohar and Marshall, p. 39.

because it cannot be perceived or measured directly; it is empty of "things." When we *try* to perceive the vacuum directly, we are confronted by a "void," a background without features that therefore *seems* to be empty. In fact, the vacuum is filled with every potentiality of everything in the universe.

We can see particles, and we can see waves, but we know that neither of these is primary or permanent. Quantum reality consists of an inaccessible wave-particle dualism, and the waves and particles themselves can transmute one into the other. At high energies, one particle can transmute into another. At the level of perceived existence, everything has a kind of impermanence.

To make sense of this cosmic dance of temporary realities, physicists had to understand what lay beneath it. If particles and waves are only manifestations, what are they manifestations *of*? Seeking the answer to this question gave rise to quantum field theory, according to which everything that exists, all waves and particles that we can see and measure, literally *exist*, or "stand out from," an underlying sea of potential that physicists named the vacuum. Waves and particles (and people!) "stand out from" or "wave on" the underlying vacuum, just as waves undulate on the sea.

Like the Buddhist Void or the concept of Sunyata, to which it is often compared, the quantum vacuum is not "empty"; it is replete with potentiality. As the Buddhists say of the Void, "To call it being is wrong, because only concrete things exist. To call it non-being is equally wrong. It is best to avoid all description. ... It is the basis of all."[20]

Finally, unlike the classical view of observer (subject) as discrete and separate to the object, the quantum view is that ours is a "participatory universe":

[In quantum physics] it is impossible to isolate the observer (or measuring device) from what he or she (or it) observes. Observers have no place in the equations of classical physics. They play no "active" role in the deterministic chain of causal events. But in quantum theory, the observer is *part* of what gets observed. The observer's body and position, his or her choice of experimental design or measuring apparatus, perhaps even his or her conscious mind, are in a mutually creative dialogue with the way quantum reality manifests itself. The phrase "It all depends on how you look at it" takes on a powerful new meaning. The observer actively *changes* physical reality, actively evokes one or another of its underlying potentials. Exactly how or why this is so, and how it is that quantum reality changes radically to the more familiar reality of everyday

---

[20] Marshall and Zohar, pp. 303-304.

experience when it is observed and measured, is the outstanding
problem of quantum physics.[21]

THE NEW PHYSICS AND THE HEALING MODEL

Although the parallels between classical physics and the medical
model are immediately apparent, it may be helpful to reflect further on
how the new physics can add to our understanding of the healing model.

- The concept of fuzzy logic reminds us that if we want to
  understand the healing model we must be prepared to look for
  and open to new ways of seeing and understanding the world
  within and around us.

- Understanding reality as comprising *both* waves *and* particles,
  simultaneously confirms the value of the "particle-ar" view of the
  medical model while underlining that this is only one way of
  looking at the bigger picture.

- Consideration of the wave aspect of the wave/particle duality brings
  us deeper into the essence of the healing model. Just as through
  relational holism the wave interweaves with the particle to connect
  and form an inclusive and whole reality, so the healing model works
  with, through, and alongside the medical model to allow those
  who suffer to become more fully themselves. And just as wave
  connectedness is not linear but works in every direction, linking all
  in a vibrant, living matrix, so the dynamic of the healing model is
  one of inclusion and integration.

- The notion of the quantum vacuum points to the silent space at
  the heart of the healing model. This is Tom's blank dream journal;
  its pages empty of words yet full of creative potential. Together,
  the medical model and the healing model help to create and hold
  this space. Quantum field theory describes the dream that emerges
  from this space, as from the silent depths of the human psyche.

- Finally, the quantum idea that ours is a participatory universe has
  implications for carers. Although there are still subjects and objects
  within the healing model, the boundaries between the two may

---

[21] *Ibid.*, p. 298.

not be as clear as they were within the medical model. Caring now becomes a dynamic event. While the roles of "carer" and "patient" remain, there is also an interweaving of the two. The term "clinical objectivity" is joined by that of "clinical subjectivity," acknowledging a shared dimension to the healing encounter.

INTEGRATING THE PSYCHOLOGICAL AND SCIENTIFIC METAPHORS

Zohar and Marshall's examination of the workings of the human mind in terms of classical and new physics allows us to consider an integrated psychological and scientific metaphor. They propose that there are two levels, mirroring the two scientific models, which are simultaneously operative in the mind. These closely parallel what we have earlier discussed in terms of the surface (the level they say works on a classical basis) and deep (the level they say works on a quantum basis) aspects of mind:

> At one level, we would recognize and appreciate the validity of all that conventional, mechanistic, cognitive scientists have proposed about neural pathways (the brain's "wiring") and their role in the brain's capacity for information and processing. There can be no question that such neural activity is involved in sifting and analysing the constant stream of sensory data with which the brain is confronted. At this level, we probably do function like very complex computers.[22]

Zohar and Marshall emphasize that this is only part of the picture and, "That classical neuroscience, which can be modeled on computers, is only telling us half the story."[23] They postulate the possible nature of the other half of the story:

> [We are] suggesting that there is [also] a second "level" or system in the brain, working in tandem with computational system. ... This second system is very likely some sort of quantum system. We do at the very least have a complex network of coherently oscillating neurones. It would be from this system that we could hope to gain our capacity to *make something* of all the information available to us—our ability to integrate it into a meaningful whole that is the unity of consciousness, or the unity of self. The two systems, classical and quantum, would not be anatomically separate. Both would

---

[22] Zohar and Marshall, pp. 59-60.
[23] *Ibid.*, p. 59.

function simultaneously all over the brain, and both would be
necessary to account for our characteristically human intelligence.
Together, they give us important insight into the nature of human
thinking and embodiment in social reality.[24]

The theory of a quantum level to the functioning of the mind also
allows for the possibility of creativity, and the experience of being part
of a reality that is greater than our personal and individual human
boundaries. Having outlined concepts which could explain a quantum
basis of mind,[25] Zohar and Marshall conclude:

> Once we have made this connection, once we have seen that the
> physics of human consciousness emerges from quantum processes
> within the brain and that in consequence human consciousness and
> the whole world of its creation shares a physics with everything
> else in the universe—with the human body, with all other living
> things and creatures, with the basic physics of matter and relationship
> and with the coherent ground state of the quantum vacuum itself—
> it becomes impossible to imagine a single aspect of our lives that is
> not drawn into one coherent whole.[26]

A HISTORICAL-MYTHOLOGICAL METAPHOR

While the psychological and scientific metaphors offer valuable
ways of looking at both models of healthcare, we can learn more by
turning backwards in time to the historical and mythological roots of
western medicine. In Hippocrates's rational approach we can see the
beginnings of the medical model and evidence-based medicine. Nearby,
among the archaeological remains of the ancient healing temples of
Greece, we find the outlines of the other model and the name of its
divine mentor, Asklepios.

Hippocrates

Hippocrates was born in 460 B.C.E. on Kos, a Greek island in the
Aegean near Rhodes and just a few miles off the southwest coast of
Asia Minor. Little is known of the historical Hippocrates, but what
sources are available tell us that:

---

[24] Zohar and Marshall, *ibid.*, pp. 59-60.
[25] Marshall and Zohar, pp. 299-301.
[26] Zohar, p. 218.

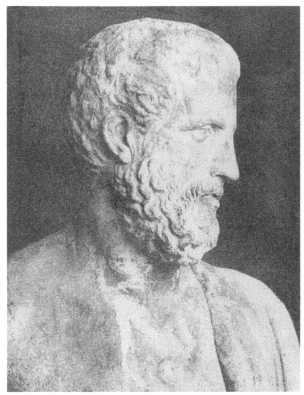

Hippocrates, the founder of Western medicine, was born in 460
B.C.E. on the Greek island of Kos, which was also the location of
his famous medical school.

[He] was an approximate contemporary of Socrates (later sources
date his birth more precisely, usually to 460 B.C.E.). They also prove
that Hippocrates soon became famous as a doctor and they establish
the not unimportant fact that he taught medicine for a fee, but
they do not provide definite enough information concerning either
his methods or his doctrines to enable us confidently to ascribe to
him any one of the treatises in the Collection [the Hippocratic
Corpus].[27]

We also know that Hippocrates was a traveler and that he left Kos
and returned again on several occasions during his lifetime. He is

---

[27] G. E. R. Lloyd, ed., *Hippocratic Writings* (London: Penguin Classics, 1978), p. 11.

reported to have helped in Athens during the devastating plague of
430-427 B.C.E..[28] As a reward and according to legend:

> [He] was crowned with a golden wreath valued at a thousand gold
> pieces when the Athenians invited him along with his son Thessolos,
> to participate in the Eleusinian mysteries as an official guest of
> honour.[29]

Hippocrates's travels also brought him to other Greek islands, for
example Melos, and throughout the mainland of Greece where he died
in Larissa in Thessaly in 370 B.C.E..[30]

The Hippocratic Corpus and Method

When Aristotle's pupil Meno wrote the history of medicine in a
text known as *Anonymous Londinensis,* he described over twenty
different explanations of disease current in Greece at the time of
Hippocrates.[31] In other words, Hippocratic medicine began at a time
when there were many different theories and approaches to illness. In
addition to these more "mainstream" medical approaches, there were
countless less conventional health practitioners. This meant that those
who were ill were faced with a huge variety of choices when it came to
consultation and treatment. It was also a time when doctors were seen
primarily as craftsmen and had no special status. Indeed, in Rome at
this time medicine was practiced by slaves. As society gave doctors
neither status nor authority, they had to earn this by establishing a
reputation and winning confidence.

> It is important to recognize at the outset, however, just how
> precarious the practice of medicine was at the time when the
> Hippocratic authors were writing. Although we may speak loosely
> of those who engaged in medical practice full-time as professional
> doctors, medicine was not a profession in the fullest modern sense
> of the term. The essential point is that, unlike his modern
> counterpart, the ancient doctor possessed no legally recognized

---

[28] Vivian Nutton, "Medicine in the Greek World, 800-50 BC," in *The Western Medical Tradition*, ed. Lawrence I. Conrad, Michael Neve, Vivian Nutton, Roy Porter and Andrew Wear (Cambridge, UK: Cambridge University Press, 1995), p. 14.
[29] Carl Kerenyi, *Asklepios: Archetypal Image of the Physician's Existence* (New York: Pantheon, 1959), p. 67.
[30] Curator, Museum of Kos, personal communication, 1996.
[31] Vivian Nutton, personal communication, 1996.

professional qualifications. Anyone could claim to heal the sick, and the doctors were in competition not only with the midwives, herbalists and drug-sellers, but also with [all] type[s] of "purifiers" and sellers of charms and incantations.[32]

The Hippocratic method can be seen, therefore, as an attempt to develop a rational and effective approach for understanding and treating illness. While obviously helping the patient, this would also have increased the doctor's status and differentiated him from the countless other theorists and practitioners of the time. This Hippocratic method was summarized in a collection of sixty or so Greek medical works known as the Hippocratic Corpus. These are thought to have been written by Hippocrates and his followers between 420 and 350 B.C.E., and were largely assembled at Alexandria in Egypt around 280 B.C.E..[33]

[These] Hippocratic writings stand at the beginning of systematic medical inquiry in Greece. ... It was in the late sixth and early fifth century B.C.E. that the first sustained critical investigations into the causes and treatment of diseases began and that we find the first attempts to define and defend the status of medicine as a rational discipline or *techne*.[34]

This appeal to rationality and argument, however justified in theory and however neglected in actual practice, is a major characteristic of Hippocratic medicine.[35]

In the Hippocratic Corpus, the authors emphasized the need to base medical theory and practice on close observation of concrete reality and to make a rational diagnosis within a given theory of disease.

These treatises show the strengths ... of early Greek medicine; a combination of acute observation, especially of physical symptoms, with explanatory schematism.[36]

Some or indeed most of the Hippocratic theories (such as that of the humoral system—that is a "balancing of the humors"—as outlined in the Hippocratic treatise *On the Nature of Man*)[37] might appear anything but "rational" in terms of our contemporary views of illness

---

[32] Lloyd, p. 13.
[33] Nutton, p. 21.
[34] Lloyd, pp. 12-13.
[35] Nutton, p. 23.
[36] Nutton, p. 30.
[37] Lloyd, pp. 260-271.

and disease, but this should not obscure the fact that they would have been seen as entirely logical at that time. The working assumption for the Hippocratic physician was that every symptom was understandable and had a rational cause:

> The authors of the Hippocratic Corpus all presume that bodily processes, health, and disease can be explained in the same way as other natural phenomena, and are independent of any arbitrary, supernatural interference. Man is subject to the same physical constraints as the rest of the ordered cosmos, and an understanding of the body, within itself and within its whole environment, provides a way to control it when things go wrong.[38]

On the basis of rational diagnosis, the Hippocratic method recommended the formulation of a rational treatment plan based on the premise of *opus contra naturam,* that is, a redressing of the imbalance in nature by the application of an opposite force.

> The commonest theory (i.e., concerning treatment and cure), derived no doubt from popular beliefs but expressed as a general doctrine in several Hippocratic texts, is that opposites are a cure for opposites. ... *The Nature of Man* puts it as follows: "The physician should treat disease according to its form, its seasonal and age incidence, countering tenseness by relaxation and *vice versa.* This will bring the patient most relief and seems to me to be the principle of healing."[39]

> Even frightening diseases such as apoplexy and mania can be cured by the application of reasoned remedies, in the form of drugs, or, more usually, diet.[40]

Although Hippocrates focused on the part, he stressed the importance of not losing sight of the whole and, according to Plato, believed that:

> A disease could not be treated without a knowledge of "the whole," an ambiguous phrase, which may indicate either the body in general or the patient's environment.[41]

---

[38] Nutton, p. 23.
[39] Lloyd, p. 33.
[40] Nutton, p. 23.
[41] *Ibid.,* p. 20.

Galen of Pergamum

That Hippocratic medicine not only survived such chaotic times and in such a competitive and even hostile environment managed to flourish and gradually evolve through time to become the dominant paradigm of western healthcare is due to a number of factors.

- Firstly, there was the reputation established by Hippocrates and his school, presumably because this method worked and was seen to work.

- Secondly, there was the fact that Hippocratic medicine became organized. The Hippocratic oath was taken as part of the ritual initiation into this particular school of medical training, support and practice.[42]

- Thirdly, and perhaps most significantly, there was the influence of the physician, prolific writer and teacher Galen of Pergamum (129-c. 216):

   The central figure in the Western Tradition of medicine is arguably Galen of Pergamum ... [this] was partly the result of Galen's own prolixity. The latest bibliography lists 434 titles of works, over 350 of which are authentic. ... It is precisely this interlocking of authorial fluency, philosophical and logical argument, technical expertise, practical experience, and, not least, book-learning that made his arguments increasingly difficult to refute. ... Hippocrates was indeed Galen's model ... and much of Galen's activity was aimed at improving on him, at "perfecting" what he had left unfinished.[43]

Until Galen, Hippocratic medicine was a craft handed on primarily through apprenticeship and the oral tradition. As a result of his influence, medicine was learned from the study of agreed and accepted texts, his own, with their constant reference to the Hippocratic method, being the most influential:

   The attitude of Galen ... in many ways marks a turning point. Galen himself very soon came to be accepted as a—or even the—chief authority on medical and biological subjects, and his views on

---

[42] Ludwig Edelstein, "The Hippocratic Oath: Text, Translation and Interpretation," in *Ancient Medicine* (Baltimore, MD: Johns Hopkins University Press, 1967), p. 4.

[43] Nutton, pp. 58-70.

> Hippocrates were correspondingly highly influential. ... The body of
> Galen's writings directly or indirectly related to Hippocrates is seen
> to be very considerable, making up more than a quarter of all the work
> of his that survived in Greek—and this takes no account of the frequent
> occasions on which he refers to Hippocrates in other works.[44]

Hippocrates's Attitude to Religious Healing

We have already considered how, in its early days, the survival of
Hippocratic medicine depended on its competing successfully with
many other "rational" medical approaches, as well as with countless
"non-rational" systems of healing. In Greece at that time there was,
however, one other system of healing which was already well established
when Hippocrates began his work and with which he did not compete.
This was the hugely popular practice of temple medicine, based on
the cult worship of Asklepios, the Greek god of healing. That
Hippocrates and his followers both respected these practices and
worked co-operatively with the Asklepian cult is apparent in a number
of ways.

Firstly, while Hippocrates traced his ancestry back to the archetypal
hero Hercules on the one side, he aligned himself with the god of
healing on the other:

> Hippocrates was a Coan by birth, ... who traced his ancestry back
> to Heracles and Asklepios, the twentieth in descent from the former,
> the nineteenth from the latter. —SORANUS, *Vita Hippocratis, 1.*[45]

Secondly, the followers of Hippocrates were known as "Asklepiads,"
meaning "followers of Asklepios," rather than as "Hippocratics," further
illustrating the close links they wished to forge between their approach
and the god of healing:

> The perfect art of medicine, complete in all its parts, as far as it is
> really divine, Asklepios alone discovered, but as far as it is medicine
> among mortals, the Asklepiads, having received the art from him,
> transmitted it to their successors. —PS. GALENUS, *Introductio,* Cp. 1.[46]

Thirdly, this allegiance was institutionalized by Hippocrates and
his followers in the Hippocratic Oath, which begins:

---

[44] Lloyd, pp. 52-59.
[45] Emma and Ludwig Edelstein, *Asclepius; A Collection and Interpretation of the
Testimonies*, vol. 1 (Baltimore: Johns Hopkins University Press, 1945), pp. 103-104.
[46] *Ibid.*, p. 194.

> I swear by Apollo the healer, by Asklepios, by Hygieia and all the
> powers of healing, and call to witness all the gods and goddesses
> that I may keep this Oath and Promise to the best of my ability and
> judgement ... [47]

Fourthly, Hippocrates writes of the appearance of Asklepios in
dreams in a way that indicates an attitude of respect to both the god
and the process of healing:

> Asklepios, if seen and reverenced [in dreams] when he is placed in
> his temple and standing on a base, bodes good for all. When in
> motion, however, either approaching or entering a home, he
> forebodes sickness and plague; for at that time especially men stand
> in need of this god. To those already stricken with illness, he foretells
> deliverance; for the god is called Paieon. Always Asklepios indicates
> those who help in time of need and those who assist the household
> of the one who dreams of him. [48]

> [Asklepios] sees dire sights, and touches unpleasant things, and in
> the woes of others reaps sorrow for himself. [49]

Finally, Hippocrates's own dream of Asklepios reveals an intimate
relationship with the god, whom he obviously viewed as a divine mentor:

> I thought I saw Asklepios himself and that he appeared near me. ...
> Asklepios did not appear, as the statues of him are wont to do, gentle
> and calm, but in a lively posture and rather frightening to behold.
> Serpents followed him, enormous sort of reptiles, they too hurrying
> on, with their tremendous train of coils, making a whistling noise
> as in the wilderness and woodland glens. His associates followed
> him carrying boxes of drugs, tightly bound. Then the god stretched
> forth his hand to me. And taking it gladly I begged him to join me
> and not to be late to aid me in my treatment. He replied: "At the
> moment you have no need of me at all, but this goddess here [sc.,
> Truth], who holds sway over mortals and immortals alike, for the
> present will herself guide you." [50]

---

[47] Lloyd, p. 67.
[48] Edelstein, p. 260.
[49] *Ibid.*, p. 197.
[50] Edelstein, *ibid.*, pp. 258-259.

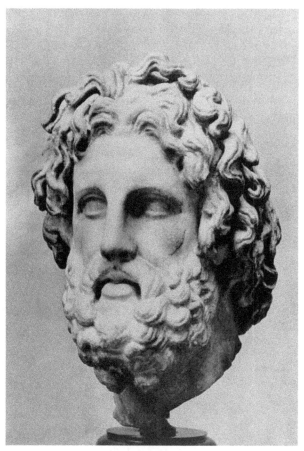

Asklepios was the Greek god of healing and one the most popular
of the Greek deities. He was worshipped for over 1000 years from
500 B.C.E. to 500 C.E..

The Cult of Asklepios

The "cult," a term which referred to the particular practice
associated with the worship of a god in ancient Greece, is thought to
have started in Tricca in Thessaly, said to have been the birthplace of
Asklepios. Whether he was initially a mortal hero-physician, as
mentioned by Homer in the *Iliad,* who was later immortalized, or a
god in his own right has been the subject of some debate.[51] Whatever

---

[51] Kerenyi, pp. xiii-xvii.

his origins, Asklepios was certainly one of the best-loved gods in the Greek pantheon. This was because he was seen as a caring god who, rather than occupying Olympian heights, trod the same ground as mortals and shared in their suffering with them. Asklepios could be approached *by any* individual who was ill and in need of comfort and healing.

For over 1000 years, from 500 B.C.E. to 500 C.E., the cult of Asklepios was practiced throughout the mainland and islands of ancient Greece. At its peak, Epidauros in the Peloponnese was its centre and there were hundreds of other Asklepians, or healing temples, which were attended by all who wished, rich and poor alike, including visitors from Rome and Egypt. Indeed, so popular and so successful was the cult that it was transported to Rome at the time of the great plague in 295-293 B.C.E.:[52]

> Asklepios was a wonder-worker, a saviour from troubles and diseases, and, owing to his timely efficaciousness, his cult grew, so as to surpass all others in the extent of its influence, during the first centuries of the Christian era. From the medical chthonic deity of the ancients, he became the almighty saviour of all.[53]

Of all the pagan cults, this was the one to survive the longest into the Christian era, a testament to the enormous popularity of this deity among the ordinary people of the ancient world.

Asklepian Healing

The actual practice of temple or Asklepian healing centred on a visit to one of the god's healing temples and a process known as "dream incubation." It is thought that the invalids who came to these temples did so of their own volition or because they felt called by the god in a dream. On arrival at the Asklepian, which often came after a journey of some time and distance, the invalid rested. The practices and rituals at the temple were organized by the priests (*therapeutes*)[54] and their assistants who tended the newly arrived invalids. A period of preparation and purification followed, which included fasting and washing in the sacred spring. When the time was deemed right, the invalid was led either to the temple enclosure or to the especially

---

[52] *Ibid.*, p. 7.
[53] Mary Hamilton, *Incubation or the Cure of Disease in Pagan Temples and Christian Churches* (London: Simpkin, Marshall, Hamilton, Kent & Co., 1906), pp. 8-9.
[54] Carl Meier, *Healing, Dream and Ritual* (Switzerland: Daimon, 1989), p. 1.

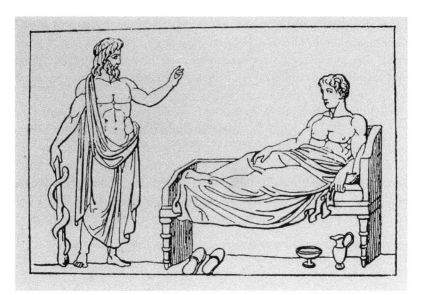

Asklepios visited the sick in their dreams. As depicted here, he usually bore a staff with a serpent coiled around it.

prepared sleeping quarters adjacent to the temple (known as "the abaton"). There he or she spent the night. Whatever dream the invalid had that night was understood as an epiphany of Asklepios. The following morning the invalid awoke either changed and healed or unchanged but perhaps with a prescription or instructions from the god. Having discussed the dream with one of the priests, the invalid made a votive offering of thanks to the god, inscribed details of the experience on a stone slab ("stela") and left.

It is easy to describe the "Hippocratic method" by referring to the Hippocratic Corpus and to commentaries of authors such as Galen, but the "method" of Asklepian healing is not so clear. Nonetheless, certain key elements are evident by looking closely at the different aspects of the process:

- Those who came to the healing temples of Asklepios suffered from incurable or chronic diseases and complaints, many of which had a sudden onset such as blindness or paralysis.[55] To the ancient

---

[55] Nutton, personal communication, 1996.

Greek mind, such diseases were caused by the gods and therefore needed a divine remedy.

• Some patients came to the temple "as a last resort," having previously tried other approaches, including those offered by Hippocrates and his followers. Although there is no documented evidence of a Hippocratic physician "referring" a patient to the temple, it is clear that they knew of these activities and co-operated with the priests, often taking part in the temple activities themselves.[56] This is supported by archaeological findings of various medical implements at sites such as Epidauros.[57] The medical historian Ludwig Edelstein writes:

> Doctors never expressly advise the use of prayers or of incubations. … Indirectly, I think, it can be deduced from the facts upon what occasions the physicians themselves allow their patients to go to the temple: It is the case of chronic diseases or of every disease, which cannot be cured by human knowledge.
>
> The negative attitude of the Greek physicians in many diseases has always been felt to be puzzling. They seemed to be satisfied with the statement that such and such a man can be helped no more. They advised against treating patients who cannot be cured and believed it to be part of their art both to know in what cases the physician cannot accomplish anything and, in those cases, to refrain from doing anything. This, no doubt, is a very peculiar, even inhuman behaviour. For it excludes the help of the physician in diseases which are the gravest and in which his help is most needed. But such an attitude becomes immediately intelligible if the physician presupposes that the patient, if not treated by him, will go to the temple.
>
> "When the art of the physician fails, everybody resorts to incantations and prayers" (Diodorus, Fr. XXX, 43); this phrase was frequently quoted in antiquity. It is especially true in chronic diseases, as it is said: "Those who are ill with chronic diseases and do not succeed by the usual remedies and customary diet turn to purifications and amulets and dreams" (Plutarch, *De Facie in orbe Lunae*, 920b). For, of course, one will not go to the god if the case is not serious. Therefore, it is a topic of the temple-cures that the god could help when the physicians could not. In a world in which the temples of Asklepios are open to everybody who is ill it need not be mentioned that the patient can and should go to the god if

---

[56] *Ibid.*
[57] Angeliki Charitonidou, *Epidauros* (Athens: Clio Editions, 1978), pp. 48-59.

the human physician cannot do anything for him. It is sufficient to
state in which cases the physician can do no more. The consequence
that the patient then should try to find help with the god is self-
evident and removes the responsibility of the physician, as it relieves
his conscience.[58]

- Although the patient may have had involvement with Hippocratic
  physicians outside and on the peripheries of the healing temple,
  entry to the ritual practices of the temple marked an initiation
  into another realm. The subsequent period of preparation and
  waiting was designed to put the patient into the right frame of
  mind[59] to undergo the process of incubation.

- The core healing event of dream incubation had certain essential
  characteristics. Firstly, it had to take place in a particular setting. In
  objective terms this was the temple itself or the especially designated
  sleeping quarters (the abaton) adjacent to it. Subjectively, this
  corresponded to the patient's "right frame of mind." Secondly, the
  healing happened in the darkness of night and while the patient
  was sleeping on the ground. "Darkness" and "sleep" point to the
  fact that the healing occurred in what we have referred to as the
  deep aspects of the psyche rather in the luminous consciousness
  of the surface mind. That it occurred while the patient lay on the
  ground reinforces this idea and links the process to the healing
  powers of nature. Thirdly, that the healing moment came as a
  dream, which was seen as a visit by the god of healing tells us that
  while we can do all we can to prepare and hold this waiting, empty
  space, what happens next is dependent on circumstances beyond
  us. It indicates that the healing for suffering is not to be found
  outside and beyond, but deep within human experience and that
  while this can be hoped and prepared for, it cannot be prescribed
  because it is nothing less than a miraculous event.

- The final point to note was that all that was required of the patients
  when they awoke on the morning after their incubation was that
  they record their dream and leave whatever thank-offering they
  could afford for the god before they departed. The emphasis, in

---

[58] Edelstein, pp. 244-246.
[59] Meier, p. 50.

other words, was on the phenomenological aspect of their experience. The dreaming itself was the healing. It was not something that came afterwards through an interpretation of the dream or as a result of carrying out some divine dream-prescription. The healing was in the encounter with the dream as epiphany. The healing was the dreaming.

Hippocratic Medicine and Asklepian Healing: An Integrated Approach

> It seems justifiable to state that the majority of Greek physicians recognized the divinity of dreams. And this is not at all astonishing, for almost all Greek philosophers did the same ...
>
> Greek medicine in its aetiology as well as its treatment of diseases is rational and empirical. About this fact there can be no doubt. But this Greek rationalism and empiricism: it is influenced by religious ideas. God and his action are powers to be reckoned with by the physicians in their theory and in their practice. ... Greek medical art is a science; it is the beginning of modern science and yet different from it in its foundation.[60]

I have previously commented on how the image of the serpent of Asklepios coiled around the rod is the only visible reminder of the ancient god of healing in contemporary healthcare. While researching for this book, I visited the island of Kos, the ancient centre of Hippocratic medicine and home to the ruins of one of the most beautiful Asklepians in Greece. Throughout the town of Kos I noticed many images of not one but two serpents, each coiling in opposite directions around a single staff. Some would argue that this image, the so-called "caduceus," is the true symbol of healthcare and make the point that this links the beginnings of western healthcare to another important and relevant deity of the ancient world, Hermes;[61] others disagree, and say that this is a later modification of the single serpent coiled around the staff.[62] It seems to me that there is truth in both these views. Although classical art invariably shows Asklepios with a staff and single serpent, the twinned serpents coiled around the staff seem to me to be a more accurate depiction of the integrated

---

[60] Edelstein, pp. 225-246.

[61] Ginette Paris, *Pagan Grace* (Texas: Spring Publications, 1990), pp. 95-105.

[62] J. Schouten, *The Rod and Serpent of Asklepios,* trans. M.E. Hollander (Amsterdam: Elsevier, 1967), pp. 117-132.

relationship of mutual respect that existed between the Hippocratic and the Asklepian systems of healing in the ancient world.

A reconsideration of defining aspects of Hippocratic medicine and Asklepian healing highlights the differences between both systems of care. It also allows us to see the potential for healing if ways could be found to integrate both models in a combined clinical approach:

- *Hippocratic medicine draws on objective evidence.* "Evidence-based medicine" is a contemporary example of the Hippocratic approach. The "evidence" here refers to objective, tangible, and reproducible data and relates to the patient. Hippocratic medicine depends on the carer using the "outer senses" of seeing, hearing, touching, smelling, and tasting.

- *Asklepian healing draws on subjective evidence.* Asklepian healing is also evidence-based. However, the "evidence" here, although it includes an awareness of external, objective reality, is primarily subjective and refers to what is happening within, rather than outside, the patient *and* the carer. Asklepian healing depends on both patient and carer using the "inner senses" of emotion, instinct, intuition, and somatic awareness.

- *Hippocratic medicine calls for clinical objectivity.* The Hippocratic carer does not get "over-involved" since this would be seen to pose a threat to one's professional judgment and ability to analyze and intervene effectively to treat pain. The Hippocratic physician remains objective and separate.

- *Asklepian healing calls for clinical subjectivity.* Because it is impossible to help patients in suffering without entering their experience with them, and because this inevitably brings carers into their own experience of suffering, Asklepian healing involves "clinical subjectivity." The dictum "physician, know thyself" applies here.

- *Hippocratic medicine treats pain and lessens suffering by intervening from without.* The effectiveness of Hippocratic medicine is evident in its ability to diagnose and successfully treat pain. This approach can also lessen the distress caused by a patient's suffering, build trust between carer and patient, and help to create a secure space within an experience of chaos. By controlling or containing the pain,

Hippocratic medicine helps to restore the status quo, returning the patient to the old order, to life as it was before. Hippocratic medicine describes how one with knowledge, expertise, and power intervenes to help another.

• *Asklepian healing is concerned with the healing of suffering from within.* Asklepian healing describes the process of holding secure space for the one who suffers. This containment of the suffering of another may enable that person to find a way of living with, and perhaps in time opening more to, the depths of his or her experience, from and through which healing may come. One who lives through suffering is changed by that experience and does not emerge to "life as it was before." Suffering may damage, diminish, and even destroy, but there is also a potential for wholeness in suffering. Asklepian healing can enable the individual who suffers to become more fully themselves. It describes a process whereby one who is limited in his or her ability to help stays with another in suffering in a way that allows healing to happen.

• *Hippocratic medicine works as an "opus contra naturam."* Hippocratic medicine acts on the assumption that pain is *only* a problem to be solved, neutralized, controlled, or overcome. It measures its success by how effectively it takes patients out of pain. Antibiotics kill or inactivate bacteria that are causing the infection; insulin replaces the missing hormone and reverses an elevated blood sugar; chemotherapy kills the cancer cells; antidepressants influence levels of neurotransmitting chemicals in the brain; surgery removes the gangrenous appendix, and analgesics kill the pain. The word "intervene" comes from the Latin *intervenire,* to "come between." In each of these examples, the Hippocratic intervention has its beneficial effect by coming between the patient and his or her problem, thereby reversing the direction the illness would otherwise naturally have taken.

• *Asklepian healing works with nature.* Asklepian healing acts from the twin assumptions that suffering is *both* a problem to be solved, *and,* to borrow from the poet Rilke, a question to be lived.[63] A basic tenet of the Asklepian approach is that the way to help another

---

[63] Rainer Maria Rilke, *Letters to a Young Poet* (New York: Norton, 1993), p. 35.

find healing in suffering is by enabling that person to go *with* rather than *against* his or her experience.

This paradoxical or homeopathic (from the Greek *homeo-pátheia* meaning "like-suffering") approach may lead to an increase rather than a decrease in the intensity of the patient's distress in the short term. This is viewed within the broader context of moving towards integration and wholeness. It demands a trusting by the carer of the profound, natural healing powers within the psyche of the one who suffers.

- *The primary training in Hippocratic medicine involves knowledge and skills.* Training in Hippocratic medicine means learning an ever-expanding body of facts and acquiring the ability to interpret and act on these facts in clinical practice. Within Hippocratic medicine, what we know and how effectively we put this knowledge into practice is what matters.

- *The primary training in Asklepian healing involves self-knowledge.* What ultimately matters in Asklepian healing is who we are as carers. Although the acquisition of a certain knowledge base and a training in particular skills is also relevant to Asklepian healing, the primary education here is self-awareness. This means that as carers we have at least begun a journey into our own suffering, that we recognize the value of gathering inner as well as outer evidence in our clinical encounters with others, and that we have started to explore ways of listening to and working with deep inner nature.

From the historical evidence, we can say with some confidence that the twin systems of Hippocratic medicine and Asklepian healing worked together rather than against each other for the well-being of the sick and disabled of the ancient world. We have considered how such an integrated approach is what is needed by those in pain and suffering. Sadly, however, this is not what happens within contemporary healthcare, where Hippocratic medicine and Asklepian healing have become separated from each other in ways that do not easily allow for dialogue and co-operation. Whatever the reasons, Asklepian healing is currently lost in the shadow of Hippocratic medicine. This is both unhelpful and unhealthy and means that contemporary healthcare is cut off from ways of working that can bring

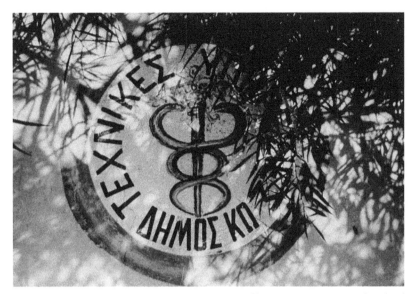

The image of two serpents intertwined around a staff is a common sight on the island of Kos. This can be seen to represent an integration of the two traditions of Hippocratic medicine and Asklepian healing.

healing to those who suffer. *Allowing that this may indeed be the case* is the first step in reconsidering this situation. Attending in greater detail to the living mythological roots of Asklepian healing is the next.

SECTION II

ANCIENT HEALING

CHAPTER THREE

The Mythology of Asklepios

Sallust tells us that "mythology is something that never happened but always is"[1] and Hillman reminds us that "mythology is a psychology of antiquity."[2] In this chapter we shall look at the mythology surrounding Asklepios in some detail because this can help us understand the dynamic source of Asklepian healing. We shall begin by looking at the story of Asklepios's birth and reflect on its significance in the light of one of the great ritual events of ancient Greece, the Eleusinian mysteries. Then, within the context of the story of Asklepios's life, death, and resurrection, we shall go on to consider other significant mythological detail.

In the preface to his book *Asklepios: Archetypal image of the physician's existence*,[3] mythologist Carl Kerenyi proposes an attitude with which to approach myth. He begins by criticizing the reductive method of myth interpretation, which he sees as the tendency of modern scholars:

> They reduce it to natural phenomena, to wrong or at least peculiar ways of thinking, to poetic invention, social norms, unconscious psychic processes—always to something else, to something simple behind the richness and stratified depth of mythology, or to nothing.[4]

---

[1] Cited in Hillman (1979), p. 182.
[2] *Ibid.*, p. 23.
[3] Kerenyi (1959).
[4] *Ibid.*, pp. xxii-xxiii.

Kerenyi's plea is that we listen to myth as we would to a bird singing, that we do not interpret but allow it to resonate in the complex truth and meaning of its own beauty.

THE MYTHOLOGEM OF ASKLEPIOS'S BIRTH

Kerenyi emphasizes the importance of the birth story of each of the Greek gods, and argues that this reveals, in mythological form, something of the essential nature of the deity: "The birth is always the mythologem that most clearly reveals the character of a god."[5] Here is the birth story of Asklepios:

> The great god Apollo loved a woman called Koronis who was pregnant with their child. One day, Koronis was spied by Apollo's white raven as she slept with a man. He bore this news to Apollo who in his rage turned the raven black and killed Koronis with an arrow.
>
> As Koronis lay dead on the funeral pyre and the flames began to enfold her body, Apollo remembered the unborn child in her womb. He intervened, removed the child and delivered the infant Asklepios to the wise centaur Chiron who fostered him and taught him the ways of healing.

There are three gods in this mythologem, each of whom is involved in parenting Asklepios in a different way; it is significant that while two are visible, the other, in keeping with his character, is present but unseen.

Apollo

Apollo was one of the most powerful of the Olympian Pantheon. The Romans called him "Phoebus," meaning "the bright one," because he is often identified with the sun. His qualities are those of clear and logical thinking and decisive action. He is the god of science, of agriculture, of law and order, and of the arts and music. Images of Apollo often show him holding his lyre. He is also a god of divination and associated with the great oracular centres of Delphi and Delos. While he can inspire terror as an archer and as a god who sends illness and death, Apollo is also a god of healing. As the poet Shelley writes of him:

---

[5] *Ibid.*, p. xvi.

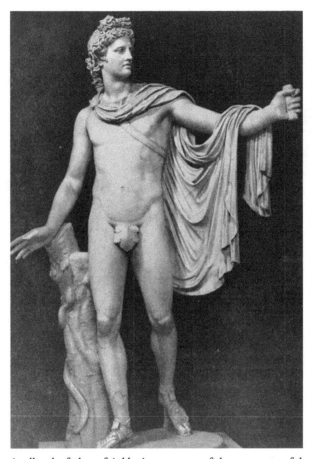

Apollo, the father of Asklepios, was one of the most powerful Olympian deities. He is known as an oracular god and was also a god of healing.

> I am the eye with which the Universe
>   Beholds itself and knows itself divine;
> All harmony of instrument or verse,
>   All prophecy, all medicine are mine,
> All light of art or nature;—to my song,
> Victory and praise in their own right belong.[6]

[6] Percy Bysshe Shelley, "Hymn to Apollo," in *Selected Poetry* (London: Penguin, 1956), pp. 213-214.

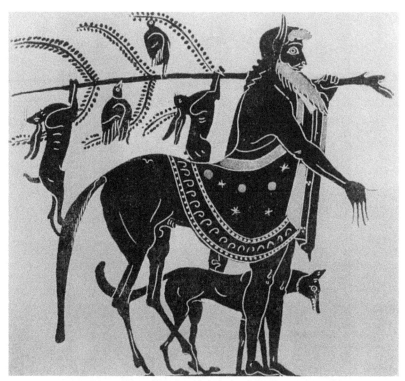

The wise centaur Chiron was known as the "wounded healer" in Greek mythology. He became Asklepios's foster-father and mentor.

Chiron

Like Asklepios, Chiron was a demi-god. Because he was conceived when his mortal mother, the dryad Philyra, was in animal form, he was born as a centaur, with a human torso and the body of a horse. Unlike other centaurs, who were known for their unruly behaviour, Chiron, perhaps as a result of his being fostered by Apollo from an early age, was a wise and civilized being who was mentor to a host of Greek heroes. As a result of being pierced by a poisoned arrow, he developed an unhealable wound in his leg. His search for a cure awakened his instinctual knowledge of healing herbs and he became known as "the wounded healer" since he could help others in their suffering but not himself. The poet Rilke asks:

> Is he from our world? No, his deep nature
> Grows out of both kingdoms.

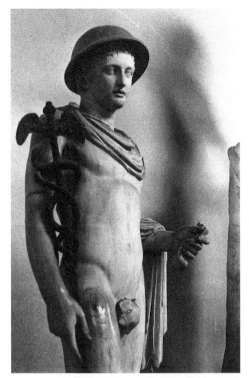

Hermes, the messenger god of the Ancient Greek world. The small bag in his left hand may represent the money needed to pay Charon, the ferryman in the land of the dead, as he guided the souls of those who had died to the underworld.

He can bend down the branches of the willow best
Who has experienced the roots of the willow.[7]

Hermes

In one version of the myth, as told by Pausanias, it is the god Hermes rather than Apollo who delivers the baby Asklepios from death: "But when the pyre was already lighted Hermes is said to have snatched the child from the flames."[8]

---

[7] Rainer Maria Rilke, "Sonnets to Orpheus," in *Selected Poems of Rainer Maria Rilke*, trans. Robert Bly (New York: Harper and Row, 1981), p. 205.
[8] Edelstein (1945), p. 22.

Hermes is the god of communication and magic; he is the trickster god, the god of thieves and of journeying. As psychopomp and god of transition and boundary crossing, he can lead souls to the underworld and back again. Hermes is the god of meeting and accidental discovery and he is at home in the night, where he is the bringer and interpreter of dreams. He is associated with the metal mercury (quicksilver) and a form of intuitive intelligence, mythic thought, experiential wisdom and complex, ambivalent communication, which contrasts starkly with the deductive knowledge of Apollo provided by direct evidence and expressed in unequivocal terms.[9] He is known by many names which reveal his different traits such as "guide of souls," "gate-watcher," "guard of the gate," "nocturnal scout," "skilled highwayman and bandit," "flattering deceiver," and "ruler of dreams."[10] His attributes include the caduceus, the herald's staff, and magic wand, which he got from Apollo in exchange for the lyre and a hat that made him invisible, which he had received from Hades, god of the underworld. Kerenyi tells us that:

> Whoever does not shy away from the dangers of the most profound depths and the newest pathways, which Hermes is always prepared to open, may follow him and reach, whether a scholar, commentator, or philosopher, a greater find and a more certain possession. For all to whom life is an adventure—whether an adventure of love or of spirit—he is the common guide. *Koinos Hermes!*[11]

Koronis

If this is what we know of the three immortals who played a part in Asklepios's birth, what of his mother, Koronis? We know that she was a mortal, a princess, and that one day she was "wading in Lake Boibeis when Apollo saw her and was inflamed with desire for her."[12] We also know that her name, meaning "the crow maiden" or "the dark beauty," contrasts with the name "Aigla," the name given to Asklepios's mother in other versions of the myth, which means "the luminous."[13] In this way a link is made through her name to the different phases of the moon, a detail mirrored in the myth in the raven's transformation. This is almost

---

[9] Paris (1990), pp. 84-85.
[10] Carl Kerenyi, *Hermes: Guide of Souls* (Texas: Spring Publications, 1992).
[11] Kerenyi (1992), p. 91.
[12] Kerenyi (1959), pp. 93-94.
[13] Kerenyi (1959), p. 93.

all we can say of Koronis. She, the mother of the god of healing and the only female figure in the mythologem, comes across as almost insignificant in comparison to the three powerful male deities. We sense the masculine identity of Asklepios's father, midwife, and foster-father, but why is the feminine element so apparently absent? There are a number of possible answers to this question, not least that classical Greece was a patriarchal culture which rewrote many of the earlier matriarchal myths in its own terms. It may also be, however, because this mythologem is meant to be understood in the context of another story in which the feminine plays a crucial role.

THE ELEUSINIAN MYSTERIES

Kerenyi argues that the essential significance of the birth story of Asklepios is to be found in the theme of "birth in death."[14] He points out that this has the "exact outlines of one of the most important mythologems in the history of Greek religion, the myth that was proclaimed in the Eleusinian Mysteries."[15] These mysteries were perhaps the most important religious event in the life of ancient Greece. Indeed, Kerenyi goes so far as to state that, "All Greek existence was inseparably bound up with the celebration of the Mysteries at Eleusis."[16] By studying these ritual events in some detail, I believe we can come closer to the core of the healing process.

These "mysteries," so called because of an oath of secrecy taken by all initiates, describe a series of events which took place between Athens and the small town of Eleusis, situated a few miles north of the city. They consisted of a ritual re-enactment of the myth of Persephone's separation from and reunification with her mother Demeter, and occurred in two phases on an annual basis. The *lesser mysteries* occurred in the spring and celebrated the reunion between mother and daughter. Only initiates who had taken part in the lesser mysteries and had then gone through over a year of successful probation and preparation could participate in the *greater mysteries,* which occurred in the autumn.[17]

---

[14] *Ibid.*, pp. xviii-xx.

[15] *Ibid.*

[16] Carl Kerenyi, *Eleusis—Archetypal Image of Mother and Daughter,* trans. Ralph Manheim (Princeton, New Jersey: Princeton University Press, 1967), p. 10.

[17] Paris (1990), pp. 14-15.

The Eleusinian mysteries were celebrated over a period of 2000 years, from 1500 B.C.E. to 500 C.E.

> Anyone—man, woman, slave or emperor—could be initiated at
> Eleusis except the Barbarians, that is, anyone not Greek. In the
> Hellenic and Roman era this restriction disappeared, and the
> Mysteries prevailed over the entire civilized world.[18]

The significance of these particular rituals to the classical world cannot be overemphasized. Kerenyi tells us that:

> They were thought to hold the entire human race together, not only
> because people continued, no doubt, to come from every corner
> of the earth to be initiated, as they had in the days of the Emperor
> Hadrian, but also because the Mysteries touched on something that
> was common to all men. They were connected not only with
> Athenian and Greek existence but with human existence in
> general.[19]

This sense of the enormous significance of these ceremonies was coupled with absolute secrecy as to what precisely happened at the moment of initiation into the greater mysteries. However, Kerenyi challenges the purist view that:

> The secret of the Eleusinian Mysteries was so well kept that we can
> know *nothing* about them. This is not true. Our knowledge cannot
> be complete, but it is perhaps more than a mere beginning.[20]

We can gain insight into the relevance of the mysteries in a number of possible ways:

* we can consider the myth of the goddess Demeter and her daughter Persephone on which the mysteries are based
* we can examine the effect they had on the initiates
* we can reflect on some of the evidence that does exist of the mysteries themselves.

The Myth of Demeter and Persephone

Demeter, the goddess of corn and the fertile earth, had with Zeus a daughter called Persephone (Kore). One day while Persephone was

---

[18] *Ibid.*, p. 13.
[19] Kerenyi (1967), p. 12.
[20] *Ibid.*, p. xxxvi.

picking flowers in a meadow, the ground opened and Hades (the god of the underworld and brother of Zeus), grabbed her by the ankle and pulled her down into his kingdom. She could not escape and became Hades's bride and queen of the underworld. Meanwhile, Demeter was distraught. She searched everywhere for her beloved daughter, never stopping to eat or drink or to attend to her appearance. After ten days and having learnt the name of the abductor, Demeter abandoned her duties, left Olympus, and came to Eleusis. When an old woman named Iambe distracted her briefly from her grief by making her laugh, she agreed to break her fast by drinking kykeon (barley water flavored with mint). Demeter then became nurse to the infant son of the local king. By now her absence from Olympus had made the earth barren. Seeing this, Zeus sent Hermes to bring Persephone back from the underworld. Just before she left, Persephone accepted a bite of a pomegranate offered by Hades. She was subsequently joyfully reunited with her mother, but, because she had swallowed three seeds of the pomegranate, she had to return to Hades for three months of each year. These became the months of winter.

The Effect of the Mysteries on the Initiates

The Eleusinian mysteries affected people in a fundamental way. Those who were initiated attained *epopteia,* which means "the state of having seen,"[21] and returned to their lives changed by the experience. Kerenyi explains that, "there is undeniable evidence that the *epopteia* conferred happiness."[22] The comments of various authors from antiquity support this view and point to how this came about:

> "Blessed is he among men on earth who has beheld this. Never will he who has not been initiated into these ceremonies, who has had no part in them, share in such things. He will be a dead man in sultry darkness." —HOMER

> "Thrice blessed are those among men who, after beholding these rites, go down to Hades. Only for them is there life; all the rest will suffer an evil lot." —SOPHOCLES

> "Blessed is he who, after beholding this, enters upon the way beneath the earth: he knows the end of life and its beginning is given by Zeus!" —PINDAR

---

[21] *Ibid.*, p. 47.
[22] *Ibid.*, p. 95.

"We have been given a reason not only to live in joy but also to die with better hope."—CICERO

"Those who take part in them possess better hopes in regard to the end of life and in regard to the whole *aion.*"—ISOKRATES [23]

It appears, therefore, that resulting from their participation in the mysteries, initiates returned to life with less fear of death. This not only gave them a greater sense of confidence and hope as they looked into the unknown future but profoundly affected the quality of their living in the here and now. Whatever the initiates experienced in the mysteries appears to have radically altered their way of seeing and being in the world.

The Greater and Lesser Mysteries

The lesser mysteries, which were the first stage of the initiation process, were held in the month of Anthesterion (February) at Agra, a suburb of Athens. They were conducted by the priests of the mysteries who came from Eleusis. These initial rites, known as the *Myesis,* were enacted on the banks of the river Ilissos. They were primarily a time of preparation for the greater mysteries and included appropriate sacrifice, instruction, and fasting for a nine-day period. Initiates could then progress from the lesser mysteries of Agra to the greater mysteries at Eleusis over a period of time (not less than a year) and according to strict religious laws.

The greater mysteries were celebrated in the autumn month of Boëdromion (September). They lasted for ten days; the number of days of Demeter's wanderings. The ceremonies began on the fourteenth day of the month in Athens and ended on the twenty-third day in Eleusis. As they walked the sacred way to Eleusis, the *mystae* (initiates)[24] underwent various rituals, including bathing in the sea, worshipping Iacchus, which is a mystical name for Dionysos, companion of the earth goddess, and preparing the *kykeon.* Eventually, the great procession arrived at Eleusis at nightfall on the evening of the nineteenth day. Even then, not all who arrived at Eleusis could take part in the great mysteries that followed:

> There were two stages, two levels of initiation [into the greater mysteries] at Eleusis. The first-degree initiation involved a communion of bread (also called "cakes") and a drink, the *kykeon.*

---

[23] *Ibid.*, pp. 14-15.
[24] *Ibid.*

The second-degree initiation could require up to a [further] year of probation.[25]

On the twentieth day, the second and final stage of the greater mysteries began for those who were invited and as they entered the sacred enclosure of the large temple, the *telesterion,* they chanted:

I have fasted, I have drunk *kykeon,* I have completed my tasks and put the objects in the wicker basket and the rush basket. Clement of Alexandria, *Prokeptic,* II, 21[26]

Many would have thronged among the "forest of columns"[27] within the *telesterion,* while others stood on the stone steps around the periphery of the enclosure. Toward the centre of the temple was a small room known as the *anaktoron,* meaning "the most sacred space" or "the holy of holies." To one side of the doorway of the anaktoron sat the high priest or *hierophant* (which literally means "he who makes them appear").[28] By now it was late into the night, perhaps already on the threshold of the twenty-first day of the month. It must have been dark in the enclosed space of the telesterion and smoky from the torches and full of an air of expectancy.

Kerenyi suggests what may have happened next on the basis of surviving original descriptions of the sacred events.[29] At the given moment, the hierophant beat the *echeion,* a special kind of gong, the sound of which was nerve-shattering and like thunder. He then called out for Persephone, at which moment the door of the anaktoron was opened. Many authors speak of the fire which then blazed forth, perhaps almost blinding the waiting initiates, who would by then have grown accustomed to the dim lighting. Hippolytus, the early Christian scholar, writes that the hierophant,

celebrating the great and ineffable secrets proclaims in a loud voice, "The Mistress has given birth to a holy boy, Brimo has given birth to Brimos! That is, the Strong one to the Strong one."[30]

What was revealed to the initiates, therefore, following the roar of thunder and the blaze of light appears to have been a vision of Persephone,

[25] Paris (1990), p. 15.
[26] Cited in F. Comte, *Chambers Compact Reference: Mythology* (Edinburgh, UK: W. & R. Chambers, 1991), p. 70.
[27] Kerenyi (1967), p. 89.
[28] *Ibid.,* p. 90.
[29] *Ibid.,* p. 83.
[30] *Ibid.,* p. 92.

the goddess of death, holding in her arms a divine child. The queen of the dead had herself given birth, in fire, to a son, a divine child. One can imagine the stunned silence that would then have filled the telesterion. Kerenyi postulates what may have happened next:

> How much later we do not know, the Hierophant, silent amid profound silence, displayed a mown ear of grain, as the Buddha showed a flower in his silent "Flower Sermon." All who had "seen" turned, at the sight of the *concrete thing,* as though turning back from the hereafter into this world, back to the world of tangible things, which include grain. The grain *was* grain and not more, but it may well have summed up for the *epopteai* everything that Demeter and Persephone had given to mankind: Demeter food and wealth, Persephone birth under the earth. To those who had seen Core at Eleusis this was no mere metaphor proving nothing, but the moment of an encounter in which the goddess of the underworld showed herself in a beatific vision.[31]

Commenting on this final stage of the greater mysteries, Aristotle says that, "The initiates were not meant to learn anything, but rather, to experience certain emotions and moods."[32] On the twenty-second day, the initiates honoured the dead with libations. On the twenty-third day of the month, the tenth day of the greater mysteries, they returned to their homes, "nobler in spirit, contented, less fearful of death and with raised hopes for a better life."[33]

BIRTH IN DEATH AND ASKLEPIAN HEALING

What is the significance of the core mythologem of *birth in death* to the process of Asklepian healing? Perhaps we may get a clearer sense of this by reconsidering certain aspects of the mythological material under the headings of the masculine and feminine principles. These terms are used here to describe psychological energies, structures, and processes which co-exist in both men and women and are not, therefore, gender-bound.[34] Although each principle has specific functions, which will become more evident when they are examined separately, it will also become clear that there are many areas of overlap between the two.

---

[31] *Ibid.,* p. 94.

[32] Cited in F. Comte (1991), p. 70.

[33] Kalliope Preki-Alexandri, *Eleusis* (Athens: Archaeological Receipts Fund, 1991), p. 21.

[34] Marion Woodman, *Conscious Femininity* (Toronto: Inner City Books, 1993).

The Masculine Principle and the Birth Mythologem

As was the case in the details of Asklepios's birth, the masculine principle is often the more visible of the two. We can learn more of the contribution of the masculine principle to the healing process by reflecting further on the male deities who had particular associations with Asklepios.

The fact that Apollo is Asklepios's father tells us that he is an important part of Asklepian healing. Apollo is a link to Hippocratic medicine, which bears all the essential characteristics of an Apollonian discipline. His presence in Asklepios's life tells us that Apollonian qualities such as logic, analysis, and clarity also play a part in Asklepian healing. It also makes a link between Asklepian healing and the Apollonian practice of divination. In fact, in ancient times incubation was often used as a form of divination. Finally, as the god of music and the arts, Apollo's presence in the life of Asklepios points to the healing potential of creative expression.

As his foster-father and mentor, Chiron is really the key figure in Asklepios's training as a healer. Chiron combined in his person the Apollonian and the instinctual. His human upper half connected him with *logos,* but his animal body connected him to the earth. As Kerenyi writes:

> All in all Chiron, the wounded divine physician ... seems to be the most contradictory figure in all Greek mythology. Although he is a Greek god, he suffers an incurable wound. Moreover, his nature combines the animal and the Apollonian, for despite his horse's body, mark of the fecund and destructive creatures of nature that centaurs are otherwise known to be, he instructs heroes in medicine and music.[35]

From Chiron, Asklepios would have learned how to hold both these polarities in creative tension and have noticed how both logic and nature play their part in the process of healing.

Chiron is also known to have initiated many young Greek heroes into manhood. The initiation Asklepios received from Chiron was twofold. He was initiated into the healing power of the natural world and he was initiated into the path of the wounded healer:

> In Chiron's half of the world lay Lake Boibeis at the foot of Mount Pelion, and beneath his cave, the valley of Pelethronion, famed for its profusion of medicinal herbs. In this valley Asklepios, under

[35] Kerenyi (1959), pp. 98-100.

Chiron's tutelage, familiarized himself with the plants and their secret powers—and with the snake. Here too grew the plant named "kentaureion" or "chironion," alleged to cure all snake-bites and even the poison arrow wound from which Chiron himself suffered. The tragic view, however, was that Chiron's wound was incurable. Thus Chiron's world, with its inexhaustible possibilities of cure, remained a world of eternal sickness. And even aside from this suffering, his cave, site of a chthonic subterranean cult, was an entrance to the underworld. The picture to which all these elements, religious and poetic, give rise is unique. The half-human, half-theriomorphic god suffers eternally from his wound; he carries it with him to the underworld as though the primordial science that this mythological physician, precursor of the luminous divine physician, embodied for the men of later times were nothing other than the knowledge of a wound in which the healer forever partakes.[36]

Chiron's presence in the life of Asklepios reminds us that with healing, who we are as human beings and how we are with the other in the incurable wound of his or her suffering is far more important than anything we might do or say.

Through the flames of the funeral pyre Hermes led Asklepios across the threshold of death to life. In this act of midwifery Hermes himself is identified as a potent source of healing. Indeed, depth psychologist and mythologist Ginette Paris presents Hermes rather than Asklepios as the principal Greek god of healing.[37] In the one who could guide souls to the underworld and back again, in the giver of dreams, in the trickster and thief who could win life back from the grip of mortal illness, we see essential features of the healing process. The particular form of intelligence Hermes brings to a situation is called "metis" after Metis, goddess of wisdom, and Zeus's first wife, who, "according to Hesiod, 'knew more than all the gods and men put together.'"[38] This depicts the dark light that guides the soul of the one who suffers:

Metis is the name the Greeks gave to an intuitive intelligence often attributed to women. A statement like "there's no understanding women" reflects an ignorance of metis, for the path of metis is sinuous, unpredictable, and unsettling for those who have none of it in themselves. Synonymous with prudence, reflection and

---

[36] *Ibid.*
[37] Paris (1990), pp. 95-105.
[38] *Ibid.*, p. 85.

wisdom, metis is the opposite of deductive knowledge and is
contrary to the linear logic of Apollo. Essentially an intuitive quality,
it is what we might today call "situational intelligence." Rooted in
an inner knowledge, an intuitive perception of contexts, and a sense
of intimacy with all of nature's ways, it belongs to mythic thought,
where logic does not apply.[39]

The Romanian scholar Mircea Eliade describes ecstasy as a
"breakthrough in plane"[40] from one level of consciousness to another. We
have already discussed how such a move is a central feature of Asklepian
healing, as from the surface to the deep mind, or from the classical to
the quantum realm. Hermes's presence in the myth of Asklepios tells of
the need of the one who suffers for a soul-guide as he or she crosses into
other realms in search of healing. Hermes is the ruler of boundary
crossings, but the ecstatic experience *itself* belongs to another.

This is the god *Dionysos* (meaning "twice-born"), who has a kinship
with Asklepios through the obvious similarity of their birth mythologems,[41] and who was one of the most popular deities of ancient Greece.
As "Bacchus," he was known as the god of the vine and wine and as the
god of masks and carnivals he was revered as "the patron saint of actors"
throughout the ancient world. He was an earth god associated with wild
nature, a homeless wanderer, who inhabited forests and underground
caves. He was often represented as the dark and shadow side of Apollo
for, just as Apollo was associated with the day and sunlight and portrayed
as calm, dignified, and distant, Dionysos was associated with the night
and moonlight and portrayed as wild, chaotic, and accessible. Apollo was
close to the abstract and formal consciousness of the mind, whereas
Dionysos was linked with the emotional and experiential consciousness
of the body.[42] This connection between the two deities was made explicit
at Delphi, which was dedicated to Apollo in the summer months and to
Dionysos in the winter.

Meier proposes that Dionysian ecstasy has features in common with
the experience of healing:

---

[39] *Ibid.*, pp. 84-85.
[40] Mircea Eliade, *Shamanism: Archaic Techniques of Ecstasy* (London, UK: Arkana,
1989), p. 73.
[41] Kerenyi (1959), pp. xviii-xx.
[42] Paris (1990), p. 17.

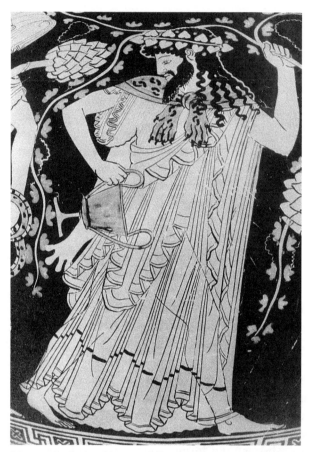

Dionysos is depicted here with his characteristic drinking cup in one hand and a vine in the other. The ivy crown and panther's cloak emphasize his closeness to nature and wild things.

It can therefore be concluded without straining the evidence that the mitigated Dionysian orgy, the "sober drunkenness" *(methé néphalios),* or intoxication of the soul, on the one hand, and music, representing the Apollonian transformation of Eros, on the other, belonged to the mantic [prophetic] nature of incubation. The erotic function here had an exclusively lyric significance and thus brought healing.[43]

---

[43] Meier (1989), pp. 71-73.

However, ecstasy may also be a terrifying experience[44] and Dionysos could all too easily overwhelm and destroy. The wild power of nature that Dionysos represents can also be destructive and needs containment to channel its raw energy. In the rites of Asklepian healing and the Eleusinian mysteries this took the form of careful preparation, often over a prolonged period of time, the specific format of the ritual event itself, and the constant attention before, during, and afterwards of priests and priestesses who "acted like therapists-guides-professors."[45] There is a warning here. The process of Asklepian healing should neither be taken for granted nor viewed romantically. It is a serious business that needs as much training, preparation, supervision, and containment as did these ancient rites. If we ignore this warning, we are in danger, as Jung says, "of going digging for an artesian well and coming across a volcano."[46]

The Feminine Principle and the Birth Mythologem

We have already considered how Koronis's "dark beauty," like the dark face of the moon, reveals the presence of the feminine principle in the story of Asklepios's birth by its very absence. Although certain aspects of the feminine principle have already been encountered in our reflections on Chiron, Hermes, and Dionysos's connectedness to the body, to nature, and to the underworld depths of soul, we can learn more about this by looking again at the Eleusinian mysteries.

As well as sharing the mythologem of "birth in death," there is evidence of objective and deliberate links between the Asklepian and the Eleusinian traditions. Depth psychologist Carl Meier mentions how inscriptions at Epidauros speak of "hierophants," that is the initiating priests of Eleusis, participating in the Epidaurian healing rituals. He also cites Aristides, a writer and devotee of Asklepios, as saying that Asklepios always bade him sacrifice to the Eleusinian goddesses and he describes how Demeter was worshipped as a healing goddess in the Asklepians at Pergamum and Kos. Meier also quotes an epigram by an ancient author, Antiphilus, which demonstrates how initiation into the Eleusinian mysteries was, for some, itself a healing event:

---

[44] G. Wasson, C. Ruck, and A. Hoffman, *The Road to Eleusis: Unveiling the Secret of the Mysteries* (New York: Harcourt Brace Jovanovich, 1978), p. 21, cited in Paris (1990), p. 16.

[45] *Ibid.*, p. 16.

[46] Carl G. Jung, cited in Peter Martin, *The Experiment in Depth* (London: Routledge & Kegan Paul, 1955), p. 207.

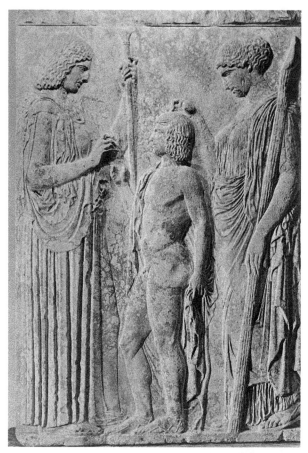

The goddesses Demeter and her daughter Persephone give the
mortal Triptolemus the gift of grain. He in turn goes out into
the world and shares this gift with the rest of mankind. If
Triptolemus represents those who were initiated at Eleusis, the
grain, as an image of life born in death, speaks of the Eleusinian
mysteries themselves.

My staff guided me to the temple uninitiated not only in the
mysteries but also in daylight. The goddess initiated me into both,
and on that night I knew that my eyes as well as my soul had been
purged of night. I went back to Athens without a staff, proclaiming
the holiness of the mysteries of Demeter more clearly with my eyes
than my tongue.[47]

---

[47] Meier (1989), pp. 108-110.

Medical historians Ludwig and Emma Edelstein point out that when Asklepios first arrived in Athens in the fifth century B.C.E., he is said to have taken up his abode in the temple of the goddesses of Eleusis and not, as one might have expected, in the temple of his father Apollo.[48] Perhaps most significantly of all, however, is the detail from Kerenyi that Asklepios was said to have been initiated into the mysteries himself. The god of healing was himself an *epopteia* and in his honour the *Epidauria,* that is the Epidaurian rites, were incorporated into the ceremonies of the greater mysteries on the eighteenth day.[49]

Such evidence points to clear connections between the ancient rites of Asklepian healing and the Eleusinian mysteries. But what are we to make of this? And what is the relevance of this to the role of the feminine principle in the healing process? The Edelsteins offer the following explanation:

> The only ancient worship characterized by an experience other than that of this world was the cult of Eleusis. Asklepios, by allying himself with Demeter, by joining together this world and the other, gave to his worship a significance far beyond that of a merely materialistic healing cult.[50]

The alignment of Asklepian healing with the Eleusinian mysteries was a way of making explicit what was implicit in the Asklepian rite and of leading the one who suffered deeper into the mystery of healing. It is as though Asklepios was saying, "You have had the healing. Now, *to realize more fully the source of this healing,* turn to the Goddess." Perhaps this is what Kerenyi means when he writes:

> The rites of Eleusis lead us to still greater depths than those of Epidauros. The way was the same, but the sick man who found health at Epidauros turned back sooner than the Eleusinian initiate who made his way to the Queen of the Underworld.[51]

The Eleusinian mysteries were an initiation into the feminine principle of healing and this was true for both men and women alike.

> [Therefore] this was a true *visit,* a *visitatio,* for which the Greek word is *theoria,* and the relationship of men and women to the person visited and beheld was the same. ... This duality—the scission of

---

[48] Edelstein (1945), p. 127.
[49] Kerenyi (1959), p. 39.
[50] Edelstein (1945), p. 128-129.
[51] Kerenyi (1967), pp. 40-41.

the Mother into "mother and daughter"—opened up a vision of the *feminine source of life,* a common source of life for men and women alike, just as the ear of grain had opened up a vision into the "abyss of the seed."[52]

In the final analysis, although we can talk "about" the feminine principle and the part it plays in the healing process in general terms, it is not possible to define it more precisely. This "talking about" is akin to walking around the perimeter of an Asklepian temple. Perhaps what we can say is that whereas the masculine principle helps create the space and facilitates the process of healing, the feminine principle *is* that space, that openness to the source of healing. All life comes through the feminine and the Mysteries of Eleusis, echoed in the birth of Asklepios, speak of healing as the miraculous possibility of new life in the most impossible of places: the birth of a divine child in the realm of death. The silence of the initiated, those who had attained *epopteia,* seems like the only possible response.

THE MYTHOLOGY OF ASKLEPIOS'S LIFE, DEATH AND REBIRTH

The Roman poet Ovid continues the story from the point where the newborn Asklepios has been delivered to Chiron in his cave:

> The centaur, meanwhile, was delighted at having the son of a god as his ward, and was rejoicing in the honour and responsibility it brought him: when suddenly his daughter appeared, her red-gold hair streaming over her shoulders. This daughter was his child by the nymph Charlico, who was called Ocyrhoe, after the racing stream on whose banks she had been born. She had not been content merely to learn her father's arts, but could reveal in prophecy the secrets of the fates.
>
> So now the prophetic frenzy gripped her mind, and the god's presence set her breast aglow. She looked upon the babe, and said: "Grow and prosper, my child, you who are destined to bring health to all the world. Often mortal men will owe their lives to you, and you will be granted the right to rescue those who are already dead; till, in one case, you will incur the god's displeasure by daring to do so, and will be prevented by your grandfather's bolt from ever again bestowing such a boon. From an immortal god you will be reduced to a lifeless corpse, but later, from being a corpse, you will be raised up to be a god again, and will twice renew your destiny."[53]

---

[52] *Ibid.,* pp. 146-147.

[53] Ovid, *Metamorphoses,* trans. Mary Innes (London, UK: Penguin, 1955), paras. 623-655.

And this was how Asklepios's life unfolded:

> Under Chiron's tutelage Asklepios did indeed grow to become a great healer who knew his art to perfection. He married Epione and they had four daughters and two sons: Hygieia, Panacea, Aceso and Iaso and Machaon and Podalirius. Of these Hygieia was his favourite and the two were frequently seen together as they healed the sick. Asklepios welcomed all who came to him, rich and poor, slaves and royalty alike. He was known as a god who cared and as a god who suffered with those who were diseased and disabled. He carried with him a staff around which a serpent coiled. His healing powers came from the depths of the earth and Athena's gift of the slain Gorgon's blood. While he comforted and cured those who came to him, he also revived some who had died. Hades told Zeus that the underworld was beginning to empty and Aphrodite complained that a mortal she had punished had been resurrected. Zeus killed Asklepios by striking him with a thunderbolt. Thereafter, it was from the underworld, or some say from the stars, that he continued his healing work.

We can learn more about Asklepios by reflecting on certain mythological details from his life story. These both echo and amplify aspects of the process of Asklepian healing already identified in the birth mythologem.

Hygieia

Although Asklepios is depicted as having many children, an important sign because "fruitfulness and renewal (as in the case of the snake) are closely connected with healing,"[54] a particular association between him and his daughter Hygieia is evident in classical art. The Dutch historian J. Schouten writes:

> It seems plain that, in the eyes of the faithful, Asklepios with his wife Epione, his sons and daughters, were wholly integrated. ... At the commencement of his "career" he scarcely ever practiced medicine without the help of his children. ... The three female helpers of Asklepios, the "medical" sisters of Hygieia, are true members of the family, whereas Hygieia always stands somewhat apart.[55]

Meier echoes this theme and again singles Hygieia out from among the rest of Asklepios's children:

---

[54] Meier (1989), p. 34.
[55] Schouten (1967), p. 58.

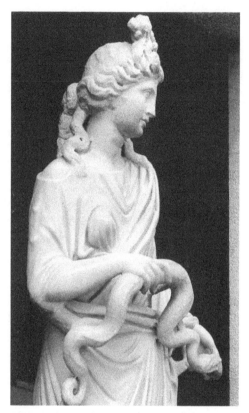

Hygieia, the Greek goddess of health and daughter of Asklepios, with the sacred serpent.

> [Asklepios] can hardly be thought of without his feminine companions ... each of whom was at times wife and at other times daughter. The fair maiden Hygieia seemed, to judge from sculptures, to have had a particularly good relation to the serpent of Asklepios, which she is shown feeding. She is addressed in the Orphic hymns as *épiocheir Hygieia* ("Hygieia of the gentle hands").[56]

Commenting on the relationship between Asklepios and Hygieia, Schouten points out that:

> Hygieia is linked to Asklepios by an essential and functional similarity. There can have been few sanctuaries of Asklepios in which Hygieia did not occupy a place of her own. ... She was part

---

[56] Meier (1989), p. 34.

of this god's essential being rather than a helper, while she, who is called "the immaculate," also sometimes appears to be his wife.[57]

What emerges, therefore, is the sense that Hygieia was not only Asklepios's "divine companion" but that she also represented his "feminine counterpart."[58] In classical art she is almost invariably shown handling or feeding the sacred serpent, which indicates that she was intimate and at home with the healing powers of the earth. Within the actual practice of the Asklepian cult, Hygieia embodied the feminine principle and its relationship to the process of healing.

The Serpent and the Rod

What is it about the image of a snake coiled around a staff that has allowed it to survive the ravages of time, antipathy, and antagonism to become one of the few visible reminders of the archetypal dimension of healing in contemporary healthcare? Could this be because it embodies the regenerating essence of the god of healing? Apparently the name "Asklepios" originates from the ancient Greek word "Asklepas," meaning snake.[59] While commenting on other possible derivations of the god's name, the ancient author Cornutus reflects on the significance of the image:

> Asklepios derived his name from healing soothingly and from deferring the withering that comes with death. For this reason, therefore, they give him a serpent as an attribute, indicating a process similar to the serpent in that they, as it were, grow young again after illnesses and slough off old age; also because the serpent is a sign of attention, much of which is required in medical treatments. The staff also seems to be a symbol of some similar thing.[60]

If we consider the two components of the image separately, we may learn more. Firstly, in regard to the serpent, Schouten writes:

> The serpent has always stood for two diametrically opposed ideas, namely as the foe of mankind and the symbol of evil on the one hand, and as man's protector and saviour in disease and distress on the other. In Paradise the cunning tempter of Eve is cursed as the arch-enemy of man. But the Jews also knew the "serpent of brass" made by Moses in the wilderness as a cure for snake-bite. These

---

[57] Schouten (1967), p. 58.

[58] (1959), p. 56.

[59] S. Kasas and R. Struckmann, *Important Medical Centres in Antiquity: Epidauros and Corinth* (Athens: Editions Kasas, 1990), p. 19.

[60] Edelstein (1945), p. 13.

contradictory roles attributed to the serpent derive from the ancient
conception of the serpent as the embodiment of the mystery of the
one absolute life on earth, which entails a continual dying and
resurrection.[61]

> To ancient man, the holy serpent was the most characteristic animal
> on earth. Owing to its close associations with the earth and its
> choice of habitat in caves and crevices, the serpent became pre-
> eminently the animal of the underworld and of the realm of the
> dead. ... Serpent oracles and earth oracles are fundamentally the
> same. ... As a chthonic [underworld] being, the serpent, by virtue
> of its mantic [prophetic] abilities—again derived from the earth—
> could prescribe for the sick. Essentially, therefore, the serpent in
> the eyes of the Ancients was not so much a symbol of the medical
> art as the healer himself.
>   Asklepios's serpent which, coiled around his staff, symbolises
> medicine to this day, is the snake whose home was deep down in
> the underworld, where Asklepios himself dwelt because, according
> to the ancient view, it was precisely in the realm of the dead that
> the mystery of life and recovery lay hidden. ... The serpent stood
> for the life of the earth in its totality; that is to say, life, dying and
> rising from the dead; hence its being sometimes cursed as the arch-
> enemy of man, sometimes venerated as the great and divine saviour.
> ... The serpent of Asklepios was recognized in ancient times as the
> chthonic being which was the earthly animal and at the same time
> the symbol of the living earth.[62]

This idea of the serpent as "the embodiment of the mystery of the one
absolute life on earth, which entails a continual dying and resurrection"
is crucial to an understanding of the healing process. Like the snake,
healing is also paradoxical. Healing means "becoming whole," but this
does not always mean "recovering" or "getting better." Healing means
becoming more completely who we are, and includes an opening to that
which Meister Eckhart calls the "great underground river"[63] that winds its
way through the roots of our being. As we are healed, we do not nor can
we know which way that river will turn on the far side of the horizon. For
some this will be back into everyday life. For others it will be into death,
where, in Kreinheder's phrase, "Death is the final healing."[64]

---

[61] Schouten (1967), pp. 3-4.

[62] *Ibid.*, pp. 35-39.

[63] Cited in *Meditations with Meister Eckhart*, ed. Matthew Fox (Santa Fe: Bear &
Co., 1983), p. 16.

[64] Albert Kreinheder, *Body and Soul: The Other Side of Illness* (Toronto: Inner City
Books, 1991), p. 108.

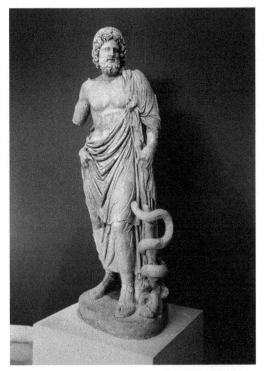

The serpent of Asklepios coils around the rod from the ground up, just as the ancients believed that dreams ascended from the depths of the earth.

With regard to the staff, Schouten writes:

> Like the serpent, the staff is a symbol of resurrection and, therefore, also of healing. The rod or branch of a tree (it is often a rough branch which the divine physician holds in his hand, sometimes still carrying a few leaves) symbolises the mystery of plant growth, thereby also representing the secret of the living earth, embodying both death and resurrection from death and thus being imperishable. … The staff … incorporates, according to the Ancients, the primeval force of the earth and is therefore magical; a magic wand, in fact, by virtue of which it performs its salutary task. … As a magical rod it is similar to that carried by Hermes who, by means of it, rescued the dead from the grave and awakened sleepers.[65]

---

[65] Schouten (1967), p. 41.

What emerges from Schouten's reflections is a sense of the serpent and staff as two images of the same phenomenon:

> The serpent and the staff, which were initially conceived of as separate entities in the effigies of Asklepios, ... were both chthonic symbols representing the same thing, that is the life of the earth, a fact which received further emphasis by their union in one symbol. ... We must therefore look upon the rod-and-serpent of Asklepios as a duplication of the emblem of the living earth.[66]

The chthonic underworld of nature is also a metaphor for the unconscious. The upward thrust of the sprouting staff from the dark earth and the ascent of the serpent through its branches could also be seen as an image of an individual's coming into the light of consciousness. Meier offers this interpretation when he says that, "The serpent climbing up the tree symbolises the process of becoming conscious."[67] Being healed and becoming conscious are part of the same process. Perhaps this is what poet the D. H. Lawrence means when he writes that:

> the wounds of the soul take a long, long time, only
>   time can help
> and patience, and a certain difficult repentance
> long, difficult repentance, realization of life's mistake and
>   the freeing oneself
> from the endless repetition of the mistake
> which mankind at large has chosen to sanctify.[68]

The Gorgon's Blood

The theme of ambivalence in healing and nature is implicit in the detail that Asklepios used the Gorgon's blood to heal. The Gorgons represent a very different aspect of nature from that of a nurturing "earthmother." These were three terrifying female monsters, part of the original generation of ancient Greek divinities, which lived in the far west, near to the realm of the dead.

> [They] had golden wings, but their hands were made of brass. They had mighty tusks like a boar's, and their heads and bodies were girdled with serpents. If anyone looked at the terrible face of a Gorgon, his breath left him, and on the spot he was turned to stone.[69]

[66] *Ibid.*, pp. 41-42.
[67] Meier (1989), p. 68.
[68] D. H. Lawrence, *D.H. Lawrence: Complete Poems* (London: Penguin, 1993), p. 620.
[69] Carl Kerenyi, *The Gods of the Greeks* (New York: Thames and Hudson, 1951), p. 49.

The best known of the Gorgons was Medusa, who was also the most vulnerable because she was mortal. It is told that:

> Medusa enraged Athena by comparing her beauty to hers. The mighty goddess then sent the hero Perseus to kill the monster. He succeeded in doing this with the help of Hermes's winged sandals and advice from Athena to never look Medusa in the eye. Using his shield like a mirror, Perseus waited for Medusa to fall asleep and then cut off her head. When he brought the head back to Athena she affixed it to her shield where it retained its power. She also gave the Gorgon's blood to Asklepios to use in his healing arts. Meanwhile, the dead Medusa descended to the underworld where she appeared as a disembodied head and frightened the shades.

Kerenyi draws links between Medusa and Persephone and tells how Persephone used to send "the Gorgon's head, the 'gigantic shape of fear,' to meet those who seek to invade her underworld. This head is, in a [sense], the other aspect of the beautiful Persephone."[70] From this, we can see the Gorgons, and in particular Medusa, as representing the "negative mother" figure, that is the destructive powers that also abide in nature.

But what is the relevance of this to our exploration of the process of healing? A comment from the ancient author Apollodorus's version of the Asklepian myth points towards a possible answer:

> Having become a surgeon, and carried the art to a great pitch, he [Asklepios] not only prevented some from dying, but even raised up the dead; for he received from Athena the blood that flowed from the veins of the Gorgon, and while he used the blood that flowed from her left side for the bane of mankind, he used the blood that flowed from her right side for salvation, and by that means he raised the dead.[71]

In other words, Asklepios, like his father Apollo, had the power to inflict as well heal illness. The Apollonian dictum "He who wounds heals" also applied to him. This highlights the homeopathic principle at the core of Asklepian healing and suggests that the healing of suffering can be found only by facing and entering the dark abyss of the wound itself. It also suggests that working with nature to bring healing does not simply mean drawing on its nurturing and regenerative properties but allows

---

[70] *Ibid.*, p. 49.
[71] Edelstein (1945), pp. 8-9.

for the possibility that the process may include breakdown and death. We are reminded here that Asklepios, like his emblem the serpent, and like the god Dionysos, is neither a simple nor a unidimensional figure. He is as complex, paradoxical, and ruthless in pursuit of healing as is nature herself.

Although terrifying and awful, the dark and destructive aspects of nature are not "evil." Just as night with day, or death with life, so these forces also have their place in the process of healing. Mythologist Joseph Campbell tells of "the Black Goddess Kali, the terrible one of many names, 'difficult to approach,' whose stomach is a void and so can never be filled, and whose womb is giving birth forever to all things."[72]

The unfathomable black abyss and the healing space are, therefore, two sides of the same great cycle of life. These images bring us back to the opening to the underworld in the Eleusinian mysteries and to the *temenos* or "sacred space" of the Asklepian temple. They remind us again that respect, care, and ritual containment are essential as we approach the mystery of healing.

Asklepios's Death

Although there are many variations of the myth of Asklepios, there is general agreement that he was killed by Zeus for bringing men back to life.[73] However:

> To be rescued from death was the highest expectation, the greatest hope which the ancients cherished in regard to medicine. Its fulfillment was held to be the most adroit feat of the physician. Some human doctors pretended, or were reputed, to have achieved this task. But for the average physician, it remained a goal that was inaccessible to him; in vain, he aspired to reach it. The son of Apollo the god of medicine, the pupil of Chiron the wise Centaur, however, attained that perfection of which the others fell short through the inadequacy of their art.[74]

If this was the case, if Asklepios's bringing the dead back to life was testament to his having achieved perfection in the art of healing, why did this incur the wrath of the ruler of Olympus? The ancient author Pindar writes:

---

[72] Joseph Campbell, *Oriental Mythology: The Masks of God* (New York: Arkana, 1991), p. 5.
[73] Edelstein (1945), p. 46.
[74] *Ibid.*, p. 45.

And those whosoever came suffering from the sore of nature, or with their limbs wounded either by grey bronze or by far-hurled stone, or with bodies wasting away with the summer's heat or winter's cold, he [Asklepios] loosed and delivered divers of them from diverse pains, tending some of them with kindly incantations, giving to others a soothing potion, or, haply, swathing their limbs with simples, or restoring others by the knife. But, alas! even the lore of leechcraft is enthralled by the love of gain; even he was seduced, by a splendid fee of gold displayed upon the palm, to bring back from death one who was already its lawful prey.[75]

Another ancient author, Apollodorus, adds:

But Zeus, fearing that men might acquire the healing art from him and so come to the rescue of each other, smote him with a thunderbolt.[76]

Reflecting on these and other versions of Asklepios's demise, the Edelsteins discuss three possible reasons for the punishment of the god.

- Firstly, they propose that he was punished because by resurrecting the dead he was threatening the natural order of the cosmos:

  Asklepios ... in reviving the dead, in making men immortal, transgressed against the eternal rules of the cosmos. Zeus, the lord of men and the preserver of the laws of nature, could not but punish him because he had violated the order of the universe.[77]

- Secondly, it may have been because he frustrated the personal wishes of the gods:

  Yet, she [Aphrodite] who had killed Hippolytus was a goddess, too. Asklepios had no right to revoke the divine decree, to act "against the will of Dis." Naturally, Zeus was indignant; he annihilated the mortal who meddled with the affairs of the gods.[78]

- Thirdly, it may have been because he threatened the divine order:

  To be sure, he would not have troubled to interfere had Asklepios revived just one or two individuals. Yet he who makes it a practice sets Zeus trembling. The reign of the gods is imperiled: action is necessary in order to restore power.[79]

---

[75] *Ibid.*, Vol. I, p. 3.
[76] *Ibid.*, Vol. I, pp. 8-9.
[77] *Ibid.*, Vol. II, p. 46.
[78] *Ibid.*, Vol. II, p. 47.
[79] *Ibid.*, Vol. II, pp. 48-49.

Pindar's description of the type of healing Asklepios performed during his lifetime was, in effect, what we have been calling "Hippocratic medicine"; people came to him with their problems and he made them better. In this he was a heroic figure. The Edelsteins compare his punishment to that of another hero on behalf of humanity, Prometheus,[80] who won the gift of fire for mankind by stealing it from the gods. For this theft and also deceiving the gods in other ways, he too incurred the wrath of Zeus and was severely punished.[81] Are we being cautioned here against the dangers of naively transporting a heroic approach into Asklepian healing? These stories seem to say that if we do, there is the risk of being seduced by power (as in Pindar's detail of Asklepios being bribed with gold). The problem appears to lie in Asklepios's attitude to what he was doing. By raising the dead, his behaviour showed a lack of respect for the sources of healing and the other forces that keep the cosmos in balance. Asklepios himself was not the source of healing. Rather, he mediated the healing power of nature to those who suffered. In Asklepian healing we too do not (heroically) heal the patient. What we can do is to create the conditions where the patient may open up to the healing power of energies which are already at work within him or herself. Humility, allied to the caution already discussed, are needed by all committed to this process.

Asklepios's Afterlife

In death, Asklepios descended into the underworld and, "Thereafter he took rank among the chthonian deities, as his most important attribute, the serpent, testifies."[82] As a "chthonic" or "underworld" god, Asklepios now exercised healing through an intimate alliance with nature and the powers of the earth:

> The gods in whose temples incubation was practiced were chthonian deities, heroes who had gone down into the earth and were invested with her powers. Two of the chief faculties of the earth were the power of sending dreams, and the gift of healing. As a giver of dreams she is apostrophized in the *Hecuba* of Euripides (1. 70):— "O Lady Earth, sender of black-winged dreams." The healing powers of the earth were expressed in the production of herbs that

---

[80] *Ibid.*, Vol. II, p. 48.
[81] Comte (1991), pp. 168-169.
[82] Hamilton (1906), pp. 8-9.

gave life or death, and were transmitted to the chthonian gods who had entered into her.[83]

In terms of Asklepian healing this means that healing is not found in the surface mind nor in classical science but in the deep, quantum realms of body and soul.

Certain accounts of the myth tell of Asklepios being raised from the underworld as a constellation of stars in the heavens.[84] This detail also has a subjective relevance within the context of Asklepian healing. In psychological terminology the word "constellation" refers to a particular patterning of energies, which are evoked within the psyche of an individual in response to a given set of circumstances. Jung adapted the term to denote "The activation by an outer circumstance of a corresponding inner archetype or complex, which is then projected onto the outer situation."[85] In terms of Asklepian healing this refers to the constellation of the wounded healer archetype. It tells us that the god of healing is eternally present, watching, waiting, and ready to respond to the silent cry of the one who suffers.

---

[83] *Ibid.*, pp. 2-3.
[84] Edelstein (1945), Vol. I, p. 59.
[85] Wheelwright (1981), p. 280.

CHAPTER FOUR

The Rite of Asklepian Healing

> For the body's sickness skilful art can cure, but the soul's sickness
> only the physician death can cure. —PHALARIS, *Epistulae,* 1.[1]

A s a chthonic god, Asklepios may well be the "physician death"
Phalaris is referring to here. The first principle of Asklepian
healing is that the way through the "soul sickness" that is suffering
is found within the depths of the person who suffers. This involves a
metaphorical dying as the patient enters the underworld of dream. The
Asklepian rite was designed, therefore, in such a way as to encourage this
inner process:

> The patient himself was offered an opportunity to bring about a
> cure whose elements he bore within himself. To this end an
> environment was created, which, as in modern spas and health
> resorts, was as far as possible removed from the disturbing and
> unhealthful elements of the outside world. The religious
> atmosphere also helped man's innermost depths to accomplish their
> curative potentialities.[2]

The second principle of Asklepian healing is that it is dependent on
an encounter with "the divine." The healing of suffering comes through

---

[1] Edelstein (1945), Vol. I, p. 271.
[2] Kerenyi (1959), p. 50.

an encounter with some autonomous element within the depths of that person, which can neither be prescribed by another nor willed by the person him- or herself. There is the journey inwards and then there is the waiting:

> [C]lassical man saw sickness as the effect of a divine action, which could be cured only by a god or another divine action. ... Thus a clear form of homeopathy, the divine sickness being cast out by the divine remedy *(similia similibus curantur),* was practiced in the clinics of antiquity. When sickness is vested with such dignity, it has the inestimable advantage that it can be vested with a healing power. The *divina afflictio* then contains its own diagnosis, therapy, and prognosis, provided of course that the right attitude is adopted. This right attitude was made possible by the cult, which simply consisted in leaving the entire art of healing to the divine physician. *He* was the sickness *and* the remedy. These two conceptions were identical. Because he was the sickness, he himself was afflicted ... and because he was the patient he also knew the way to healing.[3]

> The purpose of a visit to the sanctuary of Epidauros was to meet this divine power halfway. This was no visit to a doctor who simply administers medicine; it was an encounter with the naked and immediate event of healing itself, experienced sometimes in sublime and sometimes in more realistic visions.[4]

To help us take a more detailed look at the ancient rite of Asklepian healing, we shall consider how it may actually have been for a pilgrim-patient to consult the god of healing in ancient Greece. We shall then reflect on these experiences through the eyes of both ancient and contemporary commentators.

Being Called

Leto was fifty years old. She lived in a small village in southern Crete some ten miles from the coast. About a year previously her left breast had become hard and painful. She talked to her friends and tried what they advised but to no avail. Since it had become worse she visited a local healer. He gave her an ointment to apply but again it made no difference. By now

---

[3] Meier (1989), pp. 2-3.
[4] Kerenyi (1959), pp. 34-35.

the skin on the breast had puckered and she had lumps at the side of her neck and under her arm. From time to time a sharp pain darted down her left arm in a way that reminded her of the flickering of a snake's tongue.

One day Leto heard that one of the sons of the Asklepiads was in that area and that he would be visiting a nearby town. Her hopes rose and she went to see him. He took time to listen to her and examined her wound carefully. He gave her some herbal remedies for the pain, advised her on how to dress the wound, and suggested a regime of diet and exercise but added, to her great disappointment, that he could not cure her.

That night Leto had a dream. In the dream she was walking in an arid desert of rocks and heat. A sudden movement caught her eye and as she turned she saw a snake's tail disappearing under a big, flat stone. She hunched down on her knees and peered under the rock. There she found a pool of clear water. When she awoke the next day she knew what she must do. She baked some honey cakes, packed these with some food and water and set out for the coastal town of Lissos where there was a temple of Asklepios.

> Another wealthy man, this one not a native but from the interior of Thrace, came, because a dream had driven him, to Pergamum.
> —GALEN, *Subfiguratio Empiric.*[5]

> The man Euphronius, a wretched creature ... , being grievously afflicted with a disease (the sons of the Asklepiads call it pneumonia), he first besought the healing aid of mortals and clung to them. The illness was stronger than the knowledge of the physicians. When he was already tottering close to the brink of death, his friends brought him to the temple of Asklepios.
> —*AELIANUS, Fragmenta,* 89.[6]

Arrival at the Asklepian

All day Leto traveled. The way to the coast was mountainous and she had to rest frequently. Late that evening she arrived at a coastal village close to Lissos. She stayed that night with some

---

[5] Edelstein (1945), Vol. I, p. 250.
[6] *Ibid.*, p. 201.

relations and rested with them throughout the following day. Early the next morning she set out taking a path that led into a ravine. She was glad of the shade. Around midday the path turned up the hillside to the left. It was a steep and difficult climb that eventually brought her onto a plateau, which was dry and dusty. The sun beat down on her. She walked on and soon came to the cliff's edge. Looking over, she saw a green valley curving down to a sickle-shaped beach. On the far hillside she could see the outlines of stone houses.

As Leto made her way carefully down the winding path, she noticed that the valley floor was a patchwork of small fields bordered by bushes and trees. A strange, sweet sound rose to greet her; at first she did not know what it was but then realized it was the noise of bells, lots of bells, ringing. As she stepped off the path and onto the valley floor a sheep steeped out from a blooming oleander bush, a bell hanging from its neck. It stood and looked at her. She had arrived.

The site of these temples was chosen with a great deal of care and forethought in a healthy district well supplied with fresh water.[7]

[T]he Greeks, according to the ancient writers, selected healthful sites, rich in springs, for their temples of Asklepios. The proximity of other gods and cults had something to do with the choice, but undoubtedly climatic conditions were also taken into consideration. The sanctuaries of both Athens and Epidauros are blessed with good clean air and both are sheltered from the wind. The same was to be expected at Kos, an ancient centre of medical science, and it was no surprise when the foundations of the great Asklepieion were discovered a few miles inland from the city of Kos, on a gentle, healthful rise of ground not far from a mineral spring.[8]

The Asklepian

Some other travelers told Leto that the temple was further down the valley. As she came to a group of houses, she was greeted by a woman called Cleo; she told Leto that she was a priestess of the temple and that she would be her guide and attendant. She brought Leto to the house where she would be staying and left her there to have some food and rest.

---

[7] Schouten (1967), p. 50.
[8] Kerenyi (1959), p. 47.

Later, Cleo returned and offered to show Leto around. As they walked through the narrow streets that led to the temple, Leto was struck by the many sick and disabled she encountered. Some, obviously blind, were being led by others. Some were lame. Others were being carried on stretchers. There were men, women, and children and it was evident that, although some were wealthy, many, like her, were poor.

Soon they came to the temple. It was made from rust and ochre-coloured stone and was tucked in under the cliff face among some old, gnarled olive trees. It was not as big a building as Leto had expected. Around its outer walls were slabs of inscribed rock. Cleo explained that these stelae were the testimonies of people who had been healed by the god. Leto walked forward to look more closely. On one she read:

> A man came as a suppliant to the god. He was so blind that of one of his eyes he had only the eyelids left—within them was nothing, but they were entirely empty. Some of those in the temple laughed at his silliness to think that he could recover his sight when one of his eyes had not even a trace of the ball, but only the socket. As he slept, a vision appeared to him. It seemed to him that the god had prepared some drug, then, opening his eyelids, poured it into them. When day came he departed, with the sight of both eyes restored.

Close to the temple there was a great stone. Cleo explained that this was a "navel-stone," like the one at Delphi, and that it was so called because it marked a site of interconnection between the two worlds of the human and the divine. Cleo then left Leto, saying she would call to see her the following morning.

By the temple door was a statue of Asklepios. For some time Leto stood in the shade of the olive trees looking at the statue. There was something about this image of the god that touched her deeply. She had never before seen such an expression in the face of a god.

Tablets [stelae or stone slabs] stood within the enclosure [of the Temple at Epidauros]. Of old, there were more of them: in my time six were left. On these tablets are engraved the names of men and women who were healed by Asklepios, together with the disease from which each suffered, and how he was cured. The inscriptions are in the Doric dialect. —PAUSANIAS, *Descriptio Graeciae*, II, 27, 3.[9]

---

[9] Edelstein (1945), Vol. I, p. 195.

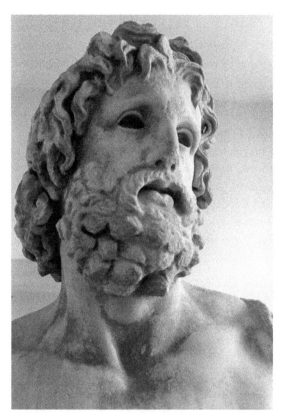

The eyes seem to look upwards and into the distance
without definite aim. This, combined with the vivid
movement, gives us the impression of a great inner
emotion, one might almost say of suffering. This god does
not stand before us in Olympian calm: he is assailed as it
were by the sufferings of men, which it is his vocation to
assuage.[10]

The omphalos [navel] stone is another attribute of Asklepios. The
omphalos, the navel of the world, is often depicted at the feet of
the god of healing. It is a sacred stone indicating ... where the first
piece of earth emerged from the primeval ocean; hence the "navel
of the earth." It also represents the place where life rises from the
dead and is therefore eminently applicable to Asklepios because,
by his very nature, he calls forth life from death. There is another
aspect whereby the omphalos is associated with the Greek god of

---

[10] Kerenyi (1959), pp. 22–23.

healing, and that is divination; for Apollo, the divine father of Asklepios, was believed to sit on the sacred navel-stone at Delphi when pronouncing his oracles. Accordingly, in the case of Asklepios, the omphalos bears direct reference to his mantic gift, which is mainly manifested during incubation in his temples and draws its strength from the never-ceasing life of the earth.[11]

Preparation

In the days that followed, Cleo met Leto each day. Cleo listened to Leto's story and told her how the god of healing, born in distant Thessaly, had arrived at this site by boat in the form of a snake. She told her many other stories about the god and about the rituals of healing. Each day Cleo instructed Leto in a special regime of purification and preparation. This involved periods of fasting and frequent bathing in the waters of the sacred spring. Indeed, Leto spent much of her day by the spring as the waters that welled up from the earth were clear and refreshing. It also allowed her to meet and talk with others who, like her, had come to the shrine in search of healing. She heard many stories of suffering and healing. Just as the waters cleansed her body, these stories bathed her soul.

By now Leto was feeling more at home. She found it difficult to understand how a place like this could have such an atmosphere of peace, hope, and even humour. Nor could she understand a new and unfamiliar feeling of inner quietness. She noticed that she was beginning to look at her own body with less repulsion and more tenderness and she was aware that she had become closer and more attentive to nature and its rhythms than she had ever been. Cleo had told her that this period of waiting and preparation would last until Leto, perhaps through a dream or a sign, or some inner sense, knew that the time was right.

One day, Leto rose early and went to wash in the sacred spring. The sun had not yet entered this part of the valley and all was quiet and shaded and cool. As she stooped at the side of the pool she felt she was not alone. She turned. Nearby a snake

---

[11] Schouten (1967), p. 46.

lay motionless, looking up at her. Perhaps it had been drinking from the spring. After a moment and with the flicker of a green tail, the serpent disappeared into a crevice between the rocks. Leto pondered on this encounter as she began her bathing. She knew that the time had come.

The priest [or priestess] was regarded as a servant of the god, and the temple was not a hospital but a shrine, so that the priest did not figure openly as a doctor.[12]

To judge from the Epidaurian inscriptions and from Aristophanes, the medical art was not practiced at the temple. The god wrought miracles of healing, and the temple had need only of priests and servants for the accompanying rites. Of these priests we find mention in many of the inscriptions. There was the chief priest, and a second one, called the Fire-bearer, of almost equal rank, and the third was a temple-servant, the Zakoros or Nakoros.[13]

In contrast to the priests in the service of other gods, those serving Asklepios did not exact much from applicants wishing to be placed in contact with the deity. When the patients had reported to the priests, they first took a bath of purification and then brought an offering in token of respect for the god. ... Everywhere in antiquity, ritual cleansing with water was considered to be highly important. Bathing was a religious magical act, in which the cleanser—the holy water—had, among other things, the power to transmit its apotropaic energy. That the prescribed baths were associated more with inner than with outer purity may perhaps also be inferred from an inscription in the temple of Epidauros, according to Porphyrius, which ran as follows: "He who enters this sweet-smelling temple shall be clean: yet cleanliness is but the nurturing of pure thoughts."[14]

The important part played by water in the Asclepieia has yet another aspect. Large quantities of water were needed to keep the pools filled. The baths, which were prescribed for incubants had ... the significance of lustrations, through which the soul was freed from contamination by the body. This enabled the incubant to have dream experiences without restriction. In this sense the bath was *oneiraiteton* ("dream-producing"), an expression frequently used in the magical papyri. ... In addition, the bath has the meaning of a *voluntaria mors,* a voluntary death, and of a rebirth. In other words, it had a baptismal aspect.[15]

[12] Hamilton (1906), p. 76.
[13] *Ibid.,* p. 36.
[14] Schouten (1967), p. 51 and fn. 10.
[15] Meier (1989), p. 69.

Of the great miracle-worker who does everything for the salvation of men this [sc., well] is the discovery and possession: it works with him in all matters and for many it comes to take the place of a drug. For when bathed with it many recovered their eyesight, while many were cured of ailments of the chest and regained their necessary breath by drinking it. In some cases it cured the feet, in others something else. One man upon drinking from it straightaway recovered his voice after having been a mute, just as those who drink sacred waters become prophetic. For some the drawing of the water itself took the place of every other remedy. Furthermore, not only is it remedial and beneficial to the sick but even for those who enjoy health it makes use of any other water improper.

—ARISTIDES, *Oratio*, XXXIX, 14-15.[16]

Fasting is the ceremony of most frequent occurrence in connection with oracles. It produced a certain state of mind, which was believed to be conducive to dreams. ... Wine was forbidden ... because of its disturbing influence on the senses. Another probable restriction was laid on beans. ... The explanation given ... is that beans were believed to act in a special way on the mind, so that dreams were checked.[17]

Abaton or *adyton* means "place not to be entered unbidden." Here we must ... assume that those permitted to sleep in the temple were those bidden or called to do so. For sick persons healed on Tiber Island, the invariable formula used was *echrématisen ho theos* ("the god made it be known by means of an oracle that he would appear"). ... Probably being bidden by the god was the original significance of incubation.[18]

It is possible, however, that auguries and auspices were taken at the preliminary sacrifices and that the sick person did not sleep in the abaton unless these were favourable. This was certainly the case at a later date, since there is evidence that sick persons sometimes stayed for a considerable time at the Asklepieion. In such cases preliminary sacrifices were continued until a favourable constellation occurred, *a numen* of the deity, which showed that the *kairos oxys* (the *"decisive moment"*) had arrived.[19]

When he (the voiceless boy) had performed the preliminary sacrifices and fulfilled the usual rites, thereupon ...

—*Inscriptiones Graecae*, IV, 1, no. 121, 5.[20]

---

[16] Edelstein (1945), Vol. I, p. 207.
[17] Hamilton (1906), p. 85.
[18] Meier (1989), p. 52.
[19] *Ibid.*, p. 54.
[20] Edelstein (1945), Vol. I, p. 290.

Incubation

All through that day Leto felt at times anxious, fearful, and excited. Cleo stayed with her, explaining in detail each step of the coming evening's ritual. She called back for Leto just after the sun had left the valley and they went together to the sacred spring. This time Cleo helped Leto with her bathing and then helped her to dress in a clean white gown and gave her special slippers to wear.

By now it was dark and others were making their way up the road to the temple. Cleo walked beside Leto. Soon they came to an opening among the olive trees, not far from the temple, where they joined with other incubants and the priests and priestesses in a circle around a blazing fire. Together they all joined in an invocation to the god:

> Awake, Paieon Asklepios, commander of peoples,
> Gentle-minded offspring of Apollo and noble [K]oronis,
> Wipe the sleep from thine eyes and hear the prayer
> Of thy worshippers, who often and never in vain
> Try to incline thy power favourably, first through Hygieia.
> O gentle-minded Asklepios
> Awake and hear thy hymn; greetings, thou bringer of weal!

With this the high priest turned and led the way along the path towards the temple. Torches burned on either side of the temple door. At the threshold Leto paused for a moment, took a deep breath, and, stepping out of her slippers, went inside.

At first it seemed dark but as Leto's eyes adjusted to the dim light from the oil lamps, she could see the other incubants around her. The mosaic floor felt cold underfoot. By now the high priest had approached the altar. He then turned and silently beckoned the incubants to approach the altar one by one. Leto, remembering Cleo's instructions, took the honey cake from her pocket. As she approached the altar, the high priest looked in her eyes, put his hands on her shoulders and said her name. He then indicated the rectangular stone basin to his right. This she knew was where the temple snakes were kept. She fed them her honey cake and returned to the corner of the temple where she would sleep.

Soon the candles were quenched and all was quiet. For what seemed like hours, Leto lay on her side on her thin mattress. She was uncomfortable and aware of the noises of others around her and thought she would never sleep. Suddenly, she froze. Someone had put their hand on her left arm. She opened her eyes to see a young boy crouched beside her. He put a finger to his lips and beckoned her to follow him. He led the way through the sleeping bodies. Outside the light of a full moon bathed the valley. All was silent. Taking Leto's hand, the boy led the way along a path she had never been on before. After walking for some time they came to a meadow, at the centre of which was the black silhouette of a mighty tree. As they came closer, Leto could see that the tree was badly damaged. Perhaps lightning or some awful storm had wrenched the huge branch from its side that now lay nearby. The boy approached the branch and climbed up on it. Leto followed but with some difficulty. She then lay down on the branch and rested her cheek on its mossy bark, which was soft, like an animal's skin, with a deeper firmness. She felt a wave of grief ascending like a spring and tears began to flow. For what seemed like ages she wept. A sound caught her attention. She looked up. Was it the wind? Just then a great raft of birds floated over the top branches of the tree. Leto knew that she was both alone and not alone. She sensed that her grieving linked her to the depths of the earth. Someone put a hand on her arm. She turned. It was Cleo. Dawn had arrived and it was time to leave the temple.

Before the actual rite of incubation took place, certain rites of purification and ablutions had to be performed. ... An initial cleansing bath seems to have been one of the necessary preliminaries for incubation. ... The *mystai* [initiates in the Mysteries at Eleusis] were also required to bathe.[21]

In most places where incubation was practised, the incubants were strictly enjoined to wear white linen bands and white garments. There is no doubt that this garb also represents "putting on the new man." It is the outward and visible sign of transfiguration, and thus also the garment of god, the indication of the appearance of God.[22]

Great care was observed in the matter of footwear, for shoes came in contact with the holy place and could not be used in ordinary

[21] Meier (1989), p. 50.
[22] *Ibid.*, p. 103.

life. Hence, … in many popular shrines a stock of old clothes and shoes are kept for the convenience of the worshipper, who returns them when the devotions are over.[23]

I thought that I stood within the entrance of the temple and that many others had assembled, just as when a purification takes place, and that they were clad in white and otherwise too in suitable fashion.   —ARISTIDES, *Oratio,* XLVIII, 31.[24]

For it was now the time to light the sacred candles and the sacristan was bringing up the keys [for] the temple happened to be closed at the time.   —ARISTIDES, *Oratio* XLVII, 11.[25]

We know that tame snakes were kept in Asklepieia, and there seems no doubt that these were tree snakes. This does not conflict with the chthonic significance of the serpents of Asklepios; most of the trees in the hieron were Oriental planes, and it is said of these in ancient texts that the sacred springs flowed out from among their roots; thus here, too, the close connection between trees, snakes and water is preserved.[26]

The main offering to Asklepios, as performed in early centuries, [was] … honey cakes, cheesecakes, baked meats, and figs [which] were laid upon the holy table of the god. … There is no indication that the initial offerings required much expense. This fact is well in accord with Asklepios's general attitude toward gifts. He was not one of the gods who enjoyed luxury.[27]

The sacred serpents in the Asklepieia were also fed with these [honey cakes], a fact which shows they represented chthonic aspects of Asklepios. … Honey cakes were offerings made to the chthonii; the chthonii were prophetic; therefore, there is a link between honey and prophecy.[28]

In the *Aeneid* (ii. 42) Aeneas throws them [honey cakes] to Cerberus, to allow him to get past [as he entered the underworld] … [29]

The patient, after the preliminaries were ended, betook himself to the sleeping-hall, and there was passive in the hands of the god, who appeared in person and wrought the healing.[30]

---

[23] Hamilton (1906), p. 91.
[24] Edelstein (1945), Vol. I, p. 278.
[25] *Ibid.*
[26] Meier (1989), p. 67.
[27] Edelstein (1945), Vol. II, pp. 186-187.
[28] Meier (1989), pp. 91-92.
[29] Hamilton (1906), p. 92.
[30] *Ibid.*, pp. 32-33.

The god of sleep, Hypnos Epidotes (the generous) and the god of dreams, Oneiros, had statues in the Asklepieium at Sicyon, and an Attic inscription with names Asklepios, Hygieia and Hypnos together. At Epidauros, too, there are many dedicatory inscriptions to Hypnos.[31]

That the incubants were required to stretch themselves out on the ground—i.e., the earth—before a cult image or altar to consult the dream oracle is consistent with the essence of the Ancients' conception of healing, namely that it was the earth itself which, through the intermediary of the rod, serpent and gods of healing, brought relief and deliverance.[32]

After entering the temple, the portico, or the adytum [the room specially built for the incubation], the patients lay down on mattresses on the floor. ... The temple was plunged into darkness before the expected appearance of the divine physician to the dreamers. "The priest soon extinguished the lights and bade us address ourselves to sleep," (Aristophanes, *Plutos,* 663). In their dream ... they saw Asklepios as they knew him by his holy images: a dignified, friendly, calm man holding a rough staff, or a handsome youth with delicate features.[33]

[I]t is important to make clear that the decisive event took place at night. The cure occurred in the abaton during the night, whether the patient actually slept or stayed awake from excitement. In the latter case it was effected not by a dream but a vision. This is further proof that the miraculous Asclepian healing was regarded as a mystery; for all the mysteries were celebrated at night.[34]

The wisdom of the ancient physicians and of those who conceived the temples ascribed the mysterious process of healing rather to the night and sleep than to the day and waking.[35]

Characteristically, this cure is sought in sleep and dreams. In sleep the patient withdraws from his fellow men and even his physician, and surrenders to a process at work within him. ... The abaton, "the innermost chamber" of the sanctuary to which the patient withdrew for the temple sleep, the *incubatio.* ... The priests were certainly not without medical training or ability. But their role, apart from deciding whom to admit, seems to have been largely passive.[36]

---

[31] Meier (1989), pp. 50-51.
[32] Schouten (1967), p. 55.
[33] *Ibid.,* p. 52.
[34] Meier (1989), p. 75.
[35] Kerenyi (1959), p. 56.
[36] *Ibid.,* pp. 35-36.

The general attitude of mind towards dreams prevalent in the ancient world requires some explanation. Incubation's effectiveness is very closely bound up with the importance accorded to dreams. Only when dreams are very highly valued can they exert great influence. ... The Greeks, especially in the early period, regarded the dream as something that really happened; for them it was not, as it was in later time and to "modern man" in particular, an imaginary experience. The natural consequence of this attitude was that people felt it necessary to create the conditions that caused dreams to happen. Incubation rites induced *a manitiké atechnos* (prophecy without system), an artificial *mania,* in which the soul spoke directly, or, in Latin, *divinat.*[37]

Equally positive was the judgment of the ancients concerning the reality of dreams, which were supposed to give men a share in divine wisdom. Nobility and plebes, townsfolk and farmers believed in such revelations. Philosophers and scientists admitted that dreams were sent by the gods. ... Asklepios, then, as a giver of dream oracles only made use of that means by which God and men were supposed to communicate. In dreams the soul came into contact with those divine powers surrounding men and the world, which it could not apprehend when it was awake.[38]

Then a mysterious and incorporeal atmosphere surrounds them as they lie, such as does not touch their eyesight, but affects their other senses and sensibilities, murmuring in the entrance and penetrating everywhere without touching anything, working wonderful works to rid them of suffering of soul and body.

—IAMBLICHUS, *De Mysteriis* (iii, 2).[39]

It [sc., the remedy] was revealed in the clearest way possible, just as countless other things also made the presence of the god manifest. For I seemed almost to touch him and to perceive that he himself was coming, and to be halfway between sleep and waking and to want to get to the power of vision and to be anxious lest he depart beforehand, and to have turned my ears to listen, sometimes as in a dream, sometimes as in a waking vision, and my hair was standing on end and tears of joy (came forth), and the weight of knowledge was no burden—what man could set forth these things in words? But if he is one of the initiates, then he knows and understands.

—ARISTIDES, *Oratio,* XLVIII, 31-35.[40]

---

[37] Meier (1989), pp. iii–iv.
[38] Edelstein (1945), Vol. II, p. 157.
[39] Cited in Hamilton (1906), pp. 4-6.
[40] Edelstein (1945), pp. 210-211.

Deubner, in his treatise *De Incubatione,* shows the existence of a
certain similarity of characteristics in dreams, which have come
during incubation, as recorded in the ancient writers. ... The
hearing of a voice was a common sensation. In the second *Sacred
Oration* he says of Asklepios: "A voice came to me by night, saying,"
and "A voice came in a dream." ... A mystical light is often recorded
as appearing to the sleepers. In Aristides' *Orations* many instances
occur. ... He sees the throne of Asklepios blazing with fire. ... The
god who appears to the dreamer, does so in an abrupt manner. ...
The disposition of the god is felt to be kind and conciliatory. ...
The god is said to be of handsome and imposing appearance, and
to be youthful. ... Sweet odours emanate from the deities. ... The
gods disappeared suddenly ... [41]

Scarcely had they fallen silent when the golden god, disguised as a
serpent, with crest raised erect, sent forth a hissing sound to
announce his coming and, by his arrival, shook statue and altars,
doors and marble threshold, and the golden gables. He halted in
the midst of the temple, rearing his breast up from the ground, and
his eyes, flashing fire, travelled round the assembled company. The
terror-stricken crowd was filled with panic but the priest, his holy
locks bound with a white fillet, recognized the divine presence. "It
is the god, behold the god! Let all who are present keep silence,
and cleanse their minds of unclean thoughts. And you, O god most
beautiful, let this appearance be to our advantage, and bless those
who worship at your shrine!"

—OVID, *Metamorphoses,* XV, 650-687.[42]

Here we have an extremely un-Greek epiphany of an otherwise
beautiful Greek god! But for this very reason it offers a unique
opportunity to note the characteristic feature of the religion of
Asklepios that distinguishes it from the Olympian world of
Homeric gods. "Chthonic" would have been the ancient word for
it, while today, speaking from a different standpoint, one might
say "numinous." These two terms cover different aspects of the same
phenomenon, but it is in any case the same phenomenon. D. H.
Lawrence suggests the essential point when he says that the symbol
of the snake goes so deep that a "rustle in the grass can startle the
toughest "modern" to depths he has no control over."[43]

Thus in the Asklepieion illnesses are healed by divine dreams.
Through the ordinances of visions that occur at night the medical
art was composed from divinely inspired dreams.

—IAMBLICHUS, *De Mysteriis,* 3, 3.[44]

---

[41] Hamilton (1906), pp. 4-6.
[42] Ovid (1955), p. 352.
[43] Kerenyi (1959), pp. 12-14.
[44] Edelstein (1945), Vol. I, p. 209.

Afterwards

Cleo walked Leto back to the house where she was staying and said she would call back to see her later that morning. When she did, they went together to a spot down by the beach where they had often gone during the time of preparation. Cleo listened carefully as Leto described what had happened and made a written record of the details of the dream.

"It wasn't really like a dream," Leto said, "it seems like it really happened. It's strange ... I'm the same 'me' as yesterday and yet ... something is different. When I was washing this morning and I looked at my diseased breast, it didn't repulse me like it usually does. I wasn't so frightened. I feel sad and happy at the same time ... I can't explain it."

"You have had your dream," Cleo replied, "the god of healing has come to you. What this will mean in your life is yet unclear. You must now make your offering to the god and return to your life."

That afternoon Leto made a small clay model of her left breast. She brought this to the temple and laid it at the foot of the statue of Asklepios. It was quiet and there was no one else around. As she stood up she looked at face of the god and bowed her head. Then she walked slowly around the temple and read the inscriptions on the stone stelae that were laid against the wall. She had read these before but now the stories they told meant something else for her. She turned to leave wondering how her own story would now unfold.

Dream interpreters did not practice in the sanctuaries. As we have seen, they were not necessary. Therefore it is also unlikely that the priests interpreted dreams. ... Everyone cured was obliged to record his dream or to have it recorded. ... The incubants were often given this command in the dream itself *(kat' onar),* and the inscribed records on the votive tablets were called *charistéria ("thank offerings").*[45]

It was decisive that the sick should have the *right dream* while sleeping in the abaton. This was the essential point for the rite of incubation. The right dream brought an immediate cure. The two famous physicians Galen and Rufus attest to this fact unreservedly.

[45] Meier (1989), pp. 55-56.

Apparently the incubant was always cured if Asklepios appeared in the dream. The god might appear *onar*, "in a dream," as the technical term was, or, alternatively *hypar*, "in the waking state," or, as we should say, in a vision. He appeared in a form resembling his statue, that is, as a bearded man or a boy, or quite often in one of his theriomorphic forms, as a serpent or a dog. Generally he was accompanied by his female companions and sons. He himself, or, even more often, his serpent or dog, *touched* the affected part of the incubant's body and then vanished.[46]

The incubants were *prisoners of the god.* ... In the worship of Asklepios ... patients sometimes had to wait until they had the right dream. ... This means that the sick in search of healing ... had to remain in the sacred precinct as prisoners of the god for perhaps a considerable time. ... The rhetorician Aelius Aristides (Aristides of Smyrna) tells us that the *enkatochoi* ("the imprisoned" or "detained ones") made a careful record of their dreams until *a symptóma*, that is, a coincidence with the dream of the priest, occurred.[47]

The suppliant was not always successful. It might be that no visitation came to him, the dream might be unintelligible, or he might fail to interpret it correctly.[48]

Asklepios healed without asking anything in return. He did not even demand that the person who asked for his help should believe in him, but only that he should be a decent man. He was free from resentment or revengefulness, and his miracles occurred in and through the closest personal contact between him and the invalid. ... Julianus, speaking of the philanthropic spirit of the god, says, "For Asklepios does not heal in the expectation of reward, but manifests everywhere the benevolent disposition, which is characteristic of him." In this respect Asklepios is a successor to Hermes, who was once called the god most friendly to men.[49]

After the [incubation] it was customary to offer up a model of the healed part of the body. ... It is probable that this custom ... arose from a more ancient one, by which, before the healing, an image of the member to be healed was hung up in the neighbourhood of the god's statue, as a sort of guide for the deity. In the inscription of the temple regulations we are told that certain fees had to be paid, and Pausanias mentions the further duty of throwing coins into the sacred well, after cure. This last rite has been widely practiced in a thanksgiving for restored health, both in ancient and modern times.[50]

---

[46] *Ibid.*, p. 53.
[47] *Ibid.*, pp. 92-93.
[48] Hamilton (1906), p. 3.
[49] Meier (1989), p. 104.
[50] Hamilton (1906), pp. 85-86.

Apparently the patient had no further obligation after recording the dream, apart from certain thank offerings and the payment of the fee. People gave what they could, in proportion to their wealth. But the thank offering which Asklepios preferred was a cock.[51]

That the cock was an animal sacrificed to Asklepios is known chiefly through the words of the dying Socrates: "Crito, we owe a cock to Asklepios. Do not fail to make the sacrifice."[52]

The symbolic value [of the rooster] is expressed in relation to the sunrise. ... Scholars were long puzzled as to the meaning of Socrates's last words ... Today we know what he meant. He might just as well have said: "The sun is rising, the light is coming, let us give thanks."[53]

They [the stelae] originally stood in the neighbourhood of the abaton, and they ... give no less than seventy case histories. ... They are nearly all rigidly drawn up in accordance with the following pattern: so-and-so came with such and such an illness, slept in the abaton, had the following dream, and, after making a thank offering, went away cured. The inscriptions belong to the second half of the fourth century BC, but some go back to the fifth century. ... According to legend, Hippocrates copied them down and learned his art from them. ... It is important to note that the men who drew up the inscriptions on the stelae took great care that the reader should not mistake the records of dreams for real events, for they invariably began them with the phrase *edokei*—"it seemed," or "it appeared."[54]

A man had his toe healed by a serpent. He, suffering dreadfully from a malignant sore in his toe, during the daytime was taken outside by the servants of the Temple and set upon a seat. When sleep came upon him, then a snake issued from the Abaton and healed the toe with its tongue, and thereafter went back again to the Abaton. When the patient woke up and was healed he said that he had seen a vision: it seemed to him that a youth with a beautiful appearance had put a drug upon his toe. —*Stele* 1, 17.[55]

The sacred animals symbolise life at the threshold of death, a hidden force, dark and cold, but at the same time warm and radiant, that stirs beneath the surface of the waking world and accomplishes the miracle of cure. The vision of the beautiful young healer appearing

---

[51] Meier (1989), pp. 55–56.
[52] Schouten (1967), p. 42.
[53] Kerenyi (1959), p. 58.
[54] Meier (1989), pp. 59–60.
[55] Edelstein, (1945), Vol. I, p. 233.

while the patient's toe is being cured by the snake is a kind of dream within a dream, an amplification reaching out for a still deeper meaning—the immediate experience of the divine in the natural miracle of healing.[56]

A dog cured a boy from Aegina. He had a growth on the neck. When he had come to the god, one of the sacred dogs healed him—while he was awake—with its tongue and made him well.

—*Stele* 2, 26.[57]

There is a striking equivalence of dog and snake in the Greek mythology of the underworld; their forms merge and their meanings as well. "Dogs," says an ancient exegete, "are also snakes." The equation can only be taken to mean that both animals may express the same psychic content. ... Dog and snake, these symbols offered by nature itself, express the same situation, the turn for the better at the brink of the underworld, and in the Epidaurian records they appear in the same function.[58]

Dogs are regarded as guides into the other world. ... Obviously their ability to follow a trail and their intuitive nature make them especially suitable for this role. These are also qualities which characterize the good doctor.[59]

Arata, a woman of Lacedaemon, dropsical. For her, while she remained in Lacedaemon, her mother slept in the temple and saw the dream. It seemed to her that the god cut off her daughter's head and hung up her body in such a way that her throat was turned downwards. Out of it came a huge quantity of fluid matter. Then he took down the body and fitted the head back on the neck. After she had seen this dream she went back to Lacedaemon, where she found her daughter in good health; she had seen the same dream.

—*Stele* 2, 21.[60]

Another person could sleep in the sanctuary as proxy for a sick person who could not be moved.[61]

Studying the sources, we see at once that incubation is for the cure of bodily illnesses alone. You might then ask what it has to do with psychotherapy. In the first place, the sources constantly emphasize that Asklepios cares for *sôma kai psyché,* both body and mind—"body and soul" is the corresponding Christian term: and second,

---

[56] Kerenyi (1959), p. 34.
[57] Edelstein (1945), Vol. I, p. 234.
[58] Kerenyi (1959), p. 32.
[59] Meier (1989), p. 20.
[60] Edelstein (1945), Vol. I, p. 233.
[61] Meier (1989), p. 51.

bodily sickness and psychic effect were for the ancient world an inseparable unity. The saying *mens sana in corpore sano,* which is often misunderstood today, is a later formulation of this idea.

Thus in antiquity the "symptom" is an expression of the *sympatheia,* the *consensus,* the *cognatio* or *coniunctio naturae,* the point of correspondence between the outer and the inner.[62]

The incubant was reborn, healed, after a visit to the underworld. … Moreover, when the postulant emerged from the mysteries, he was himself a *religiosus, a cultor deae:* this corresponds to the Greek term *therapeutés.* … Mysteries presuppose *epopteia* (spectators), who see the *drómenon* (action). In the case of incubation, the incubant would have been the *epoptés,* and the *drómenon* which he had witnessed would have been the dream; while the healing itself would have been the mystery.[63]

I myself am one of those who have lived not twice but many and varied lives through the power of the god, and consequently one of those who think that sickness for this reason is advantageous and who moreover have acquired precious gems in return for which I would not accept all that which is considered happiness among men. —ARISTIDES, *Oratio,* XXIII, 15-18.[64]

[62] *Ibid.,* p. iv.
[63] *Ibid.,* p. 107.
[64] Edelstein (1945), Vol. I, p. 203.

SECTION III

THEORY

CHAPTER FIVE

The Containment of Care

The pilgrim patients of ancient Greece who traveled to an Asklepian in search of healing would have discovered that this came as a dream epiphany within the *temenos* of the temple precinct. This "sacred space" described the subjective state of readiness and openness created by the relationships with the priests and priestesses and the rituals of preparation, as well as referring to the actual space contained by the walls of the healing temple itself. As psychotherapist Henry Reed puts it:

> [The ritual of incubation is] an externalization of a psychological fact—a projection mirroring a natural inner process. It is as if the incubant were able, by aligning him or herself with the symbolic structure of the ritual, to allow a certain inner condition to arise, which cannot be produced directly.[1]

One possible way of understanding how this might translate into contemporary healthcare practice is to consider the metaphor of the alchemical container, the so-called *vas bene clausum* or "well-sealed vessel," where miraculous transformation can occur.

---

[1] Henry Reed, "Dream Incubation: A Reconstruction of a Ritual in Contemporary Form," *Journal of Humanistic Psychology* 13 (1974): 3.

THE ALCHEMICAL CONTAINER

While the roots of alchemy are complex and deep and reach back to ancient China and India, the first recordings of this art are in Egypt, and the earliest alchemists were Egyptian and Jewish.[2] Alchemy came to the west in the Middle Ages. Having permeated Islamic culture from the eighth century as a result of Arab involvement in Egypt, it was brought in turn by the Arabs to Spain and southern Italy. The first known translation of an Arabic alchemical text into English was made in 1144.[3]

Some know alchemy as the forerunner of chemistry, but most will associate it with seemingly foolhardy attempts to change base metal into gold. In essence alchemists were concerned with the process of transformation and change. Analytical psychologist Nathan Schwartz-Salant explains:

> The alchemists worked with materials that they tried to change from base to more elevated forms, or they attempted to tincture substances to change their appearance, an endeavour that owed much to the Egyptian craft of dyeing fabrics. In general, alchemy attempted to deal with the complexities of change, the transformation from one state or form to another, from a seed to an embryo, or from an ore of little value to silver or gold, transformed, they believed, in the bowels of the earth under intense pressures and heat. The alchemical art attempted to imitate such processes in a laboratory. But this outer or mundane work with materials was intimately linked to an inner or arcane work on the human personality. For example, the alchemical fire, which is often called the secret of the *opus,* is clearly a physical fire, controlled within an actual vessel, but it is also the heat-producing quality of meditation and imagination.[4]

Jung saw in alchemy a close metaphor of the process of inner change and psychological transformation:

> In alchemy ... Jung found a mine of symbolism that he recognized to parallel the way a human being, with a correct use of will and imagination, and the assent of fate, can enter a process whose goal is the creation of an internal structure he called the [S]elf. The [S]elf,

---

[2] Jay Ramsey, *Alchemy: The Art of Transformation* (London, UK: Thorsons, 1997), pp. 17-18.

[3] *Ibid.*, p. 21.

[4] Nathan Schwartz-Salant, *C. G. Jung: Jung on Alchemy* (London, UK: Routledge, 1995), p. 2.

created through what Jung termed the individuation process, yields an inner stability and sense of direction for the ego even amidst stormy, emotional and environmental conflict. But the [S]elf is filled with paradox, and it too can create chaotic states of mind that can endanger a person's sense of identity. Usually this has a greater goal of enriching and widening the scope and values of the personality. But it also has its dangers. "Many have perished in the work" is an alchemical saying that Jung quotes to offer a balance to any overly optimistic attitude. Jung found that alchemy mirrored the complexities of the process of the creation of the [S]elf in ways far superior to any other body of thought.[5]

Of central importance to this process, maximizing its chances of success and minimizing the dangers associated with the work, was the alchemical vessel, within which the process of transformation took place:

The *vas bene clausum* (well-sealed vessel) is a precautionary measure very frequently mentioned in alchemy, and it is the equivalent of the magic circle. In both cases the idea is to protect what is within from the intrusion and admixture of what is without, as well as to prevent it from escaping.[6]

As Jungian analyst Christopher Perry points out, there are parallels between the alchemical vessel and the analytic encounter. The *vas bene clausum* is a way of describing:

The analytic setting and ... the analyst's interventions which are required to keep the heat at a level of anxiety optimal to the patient's self-discovery and the analyst's development both as an analyst and as a human being.[7]

In a similar vein, chaplain and psychotherapist Peter Speck stresses that the ability to "contain" powerful reactions and strong emotions is an essential part of all caring relationships:

The word "containment" is not used here in a physical sense but refers to the emotional and psychological capacity to hold powerful

[5] *Ibid.*
[6] Carl G. Jung, *The Collected Works of C. G. Jung*, 2nd ed., trans. R. F. C. Hull, ed. H. Read, M. Fordham, G. Adler, and W. McGuire (Princeton: Princeton University Press, 1966–70), *Psychology and Alchemy* 12, "The Symbolism of the Mandala," para. 219.
[7] Christopher Perry, "Transference and Countertransference," in *The Cambridge Companion to Jung*, ed. Polly Young-Eisendrath and Terence Dawson (Cambridge, UK: Cambridge University Press, 1997), p. 148.

and conflicting feelings, which are aroused in oneself unconsciously by others, without either retaliating or offering mindless reassurance. Such containment is a prerequisite of any therapeutic community.[8]

We shall now examine more closely what the idea of containment might mean when working with another in suffering.

Suffering as Container

Suffering itself may become an alchemical container. Psychotherapist Kay Duff, writing of her own experience of living with suffering, explains how:

> The alchemists insisted that two things must happen before the cure can be extracted from the disease: the problem must be kept in a closed container, and it must be reduced to its original state through a process of breakdown. The limitations and immobility of illness provide the closed container that enables this transformation, precisely because there is no way out.

> The isolation and lack of sympathy or understanding that sick people often endure may even be necessary to secure the walls of the container, so that nothing is spilt or shared, and the matter inside will reach the point of transmutation. The walled space of illness, like therapy, intensifies the brooding and incubates the egg.[9]

This "intensification" is the build-up of heat necessary to dissolve the problem down to its constituent parts, the essential first step in alchemical change:

> In the closed container of the alchemist's flask, the problem is reduced, broken down, and returned to its original state of disorder, which the alchemists termed *massa confusa,* meaning confused mass. What has been learned under the assumptions of health must be unlearned under the exigencies of disease.[10]

And so, what can at times seem like the prison walls of suffering can also be seen as the firm, containing boundaries of the alchemical vessel, marking out and holding the space for potential change.

---

[8] Peter Speck, "Unconscious Communications" (editorial), *Palliative Medicine* 10 (1996): 273.

[9] Kay Duff, *The Alchemy of Illness* (New York: Bell Tower, 1993), p. 81.

[10] *Ibid.*, p. 83.

Teamwork as Container

The "team" of "teamwork" may be the family of the patient with the community-based healthcare workers, if the patient is at home, or the hospital-based healthcare workers if the patient is in hospital. The most significant factor in creating containment for the person in suffering is the web of caring relationships that establish security and trust with that person. However, the containment that is created by interprofessional teamwork does not simply come about because a number of different disciplines happen to be involved in that patient's care and treatment. The container has to be built, a process which involves deliberate and conscious effort. There are certain key elements in this:

- The patient's family and close friends must be seen as core members of the caring team.

- Each discipline involved in patient care must have a clear sense of its own professional identity. This entails clearly identifying that particular discipline's strengths and limitations. Although this is especially pertinent to the different professional healthcare disciplines, it also applies to family and friends of the patient and carers who are involved in a voluntary capacity.

- Among the different professional and voluntary groups involved in an individual patient's care, there must be an acknowledgement of and respect for the contribution and skills that the others have to offer. There must also be an awareness of shared areas of care, where close communication and co-operation are essential to avoid duplication of effort, interdisciplinary territorialism, and confusion or "flooding" of the patient.

- The process of team self-awareness comes through individual disciplines meeting together and with regular interdisciplinary team meetings. The occasional input of an external facilitator who is experienced in team management and psychodynamics can be invaluable in this process. This is particularly true in the early stages of team building but can also be helpful for well-established teams when dealing with difficult issues arising from an individual patient's care.

Although good intra- and interdisciplinary communication is the priority task for the caring team interested in building a secure-enough container for the patient in suffering, the level of skills of the different disciplines that make up the team is also important. In other words, each discipline needs to be fully versed in the Hippocratic approach as it applies to its domain of clinical responsibility and to be effective in its therapeutic task. Such competence helps to create trust with patients, to lessen their sense of fear, and to increase their sense of security. These are essential ingredients in building the containment of care.

Relationship as Container

Cicely Saunders speaks of the containment that is relationship in the following way:

> The real presence of another person is a place of security. I recall remarking to two psychiatrists that when patients are in a climate of safety they will come to realise what is happening in their own way and not be afraid. One said: "How can you speak of a climate of safety when death is the most unsafe thing that can happen?" To which the other replied: "I think you are using the wrong word. I think it should be "security." A child separated from his mother may be quite safe—but he feels very insecure. A child in his mother's arms during an air raid may be very unsafe indeed—but he feels quite secure." We have to give all patients that feeling of security in which they can begin, when they are ready, to face unsafety.[11]

The idea of relationship as container is one that has been explored extensively in psychoanalytic literature in terms of the psychotherapeutic relationship. One psychoanalyst whose thinking seems particularly relevant in this regard is Wilfred Bion. His model of "container/contained" has been clearly summarized by psychoanalytic psychotherapist Ricky Emmanuel:

> In Bion's theory, the development of the capacity to think, or be curious in any way, or to pay attention or learn from experience, depends upon the baby's experience of being thought about, or having had the experience of someone being curious or attentive about him or her. In the same way as the child will not learn to talk unless he has been talked to, so the same applies to thinking, curiosity or attention.
> ... From sense data available to the baby from within him or without, the baby is faced with the problem of what is this object, feelings, sensation or whatever. The bombardment of meaningless

---

[11] Saunders (1978), p. 6.

data reaching the baby through its senses may overwhelm him and all he can do is evacuate these unpleasant feelings and sensations. The baby's psyche is not developed enough to contain powerful feelings of any kind and is thus absolutely dependent upon the availability of some object into whom the baby can rid himself of these feelings. Bion calls this object *the container* and the stuff put into the container, in this instance, overwhelming incomprehensible painful sense data, *the contained*. The container, the mother ... then has to try and make sense out of the baby's experience by thinking about whatever it is the baby has made her feel. She can only do this if she has had an experience of a mother who could do this for her, which she has internalized and carries within her. This thinking about the communication from the baby which the mother has to do, to sort out what the baby is communicating, Bion calls *reverie*. Once the mother has sorted out what the baby is communicating, she can respond to him and the baby may feel understood. In other words, the container acts upon the contained through the function of reverie and then can hand back the contained to the baby, in more digested modified form.

... As the baby has more and more experience like this, it enables him to take into his mind a "thinking object" if you like. He can then use this thinking object, this container, which is now internalized, to begin to think for himself and his own experience. Thus he begins to develop his own capacity to think and have a space in his own mind. He becomes stronger, less overwhelmed by experience, more able to wait and able to make sense of the sense data coming to him, i.e., he can pay attention to things through identifying with the container who attended to him.

Bion says that the baby's feelings are too powerful to be contained within his own personality. By being able to project them into a container, the baby can investigate these feelings in a personality powerful enough to contain them. He gives the example of the baby fearing it is dying (which in turn arouses the) fear that it is dying in the mother [and concludes;] "A well balanced mother can accept these feelings and respond therapeutically i.e., in a manner that makes the infant feel it is receiving its frightened personality back again, but in a form that it can tolerate—the fears are manageable by the infant personality."[12]

To those unfamiliar with the psychoanalytic literature, all this talk of "mother" and "overwhelmed infants" may seem far removed from the concrete, everyday experience of caring for someone who is living with

---

[12] W. R. Bion, "A theory of thinking," *International Journal of Psycho-Analysis* 43 (1962): 4-5; cited in Ricky Emmanuel, personal communication (Tavistock Lecture), 1996.

advanced or incurable illness. From my experience, however, Bion's
"container/contained" theory seems like an accurate description of what
I repeatedly encounter in clinical practice.

Those suffering with advanced or incurable illness are facing into the
unknown. As one patient put it to me some days before she died, "I need
help with this [dying]. I've never done it before." It seems very plausible
that the powerful feelings that such experiences engender in patients could
resonate with the long-forgotten and possibly pre-verbal memories of
impotence and helplessness of infancy to trigger primitive survival
reactions along the lines Bion suggests. There is a real danger of the patient
being overwhelmed or immobilized by these primal emotions. According
to Bion's theory, "being there" with another in his or her suffering includes
an ability to contain this emotional material. This containment by the carer
enables the patient to feel heard, as well as to feel held and secure. By
considering and processing (Bion's "thinking" or "reverie") the contained
material at an individual and team level and then responding in an
appropriate way, the carer(s) can begin to meet that patient's needs and
empower that individual to live with his or her own ambivalent feelings.

The obvious relevance of Bion's observations to the caring
relationship highlights the need to have more of the insights of
psychoanalytic theory translated into everyday clinical concepts in the
hope of creating a more conscious and thereby more holistic mode of
caring. This may not only increase the effectiveness of clinical practice
but help to prevent staff burnout and abuses of the obvious power
differentials that exist in such settings.[13]

The solid, stone walls of the Asklepian healing temple are a metaphor
for the containment of care. We have considered how this is created for the
patient in the clinical setting by the experience of suffering itself, and
through relationships with the team and its individual members. We shall
now consider in more detail what this might mean for the individual carer.

---

[13] Adolf Guggenbühl-Craig, *Power in the Helping Professions* (Texas: Spring
Publications, 1971).

CHAPTER SIX

Towards a Therapeutic Use of Self

T he fact that Asklepios was seen as patron of physicians (as well as patients) means that in working with another in suffering the carer him- or herself is an essential part of the healing process. In Asklepian healing the being (who we are and how we are with the patient) is *primary* and the doing (the actual practice of skilled and effective caring) follows on from this. The late Hindu teacher Sri Madhava Ashish points to what is necessary here:

> "Physician heal thyself" would appear to be the axiom. For it's an Alice through the looking glass affair. When one sees a door reflected in a mirror, to reach the actual door, one must first move away from the mirror.
>
> When you want to help a person towards healing you must, in some way, retreat into yourself to the level from which the healing flows.[1]

Carl Jung frequently commented on this theme. In his autobiography, *Memories, Dreams, Reflections,* he writes:

> In any ongoing analysis the whole personality of both patient and doctor is called into play. There are many cases which the doctor cannot cure without committing himself. When important matters

---

[1] Sri Madhava Ashish, personal communication, 1992.

are at stake, it makes all the difference whether the doctor sees himself as a part of the drama, or cloaks himself in his authority. In the great crises of life, in the supreme moments when to be or not to be is the question, little tricks of suggestion do not help. Then the whole being of the doctor is challenged.

... The doctor is effective only when he himself is affected. "Only the wounded physician heals." But when the doctor wears his personality like a coat of armour, he has no effect.[2]

To know ourselves as carers is an essential part of the process of containing another's suffering. But what might this look like in practice? In terms of psychoanalysis, Jung and others are clear that this means that all trainee psychotherapists should themselves undergo extensive personal psychotherapy and subsequently continue in clinical supervision with an experienced colleague.

The psychotherapist, however, must understand not only the patient; it is equally important that he should understand himself. For that reason the *sine qua non* is the analysis of the analyst, what is called the training analysis. The patient's treatment begins with the doctor, so to speak. Only if the doctor knows how to cope with himself and his own problems will he be able to teach the patient to do the same. Only then. In the training analysis the doctor must learn to know his own psyche and to take it seriously ... [3]

Jung's early insistence on a training analysis sprang from his view that analysts could accompany their patients only as far as they themselves had gone in their quest for self-awareness. This position is qualified by Christopher Perry when he writes:

Its invalidity rests on the supposition that the analyst can potentially empathise and identify with any psychic content within a patient. ... Analysts can also act as containers for apparently incomprehensible aspects of their patients whilst the latter gain distance and the advantage of objectivity. Furthermore, analysts can act as companions and witnesses to experiences unknown to themselves but always waiting in the theatre of life.[4]

To acknowledge that it is unnecessary to *fully* know ourselves in order to contain the suffering of another (an impossible task in any case),

[2] Carl G. Jung, *Memories, Dreams, Reflections* (London, UK: Flamingo, 1983), pp. 155-156.
[3] *Ibid.*, pp. 154-156.
[4] Christopher Perry (1997) op. cit., p. 157.

however, by no means invalidates the necessity and the value of at least *beginning* in this process. A failure to do so has potentially negative consequences for the therapeutic relationship. Jung gives some of the reasons for this when he writes:

> The therapist must at all times keep watch over himself, over the way he is reacting to his patient. For we do not react only with our consciousness. Also we must always be asking ourselves: How is our unconscious experiencing this situation? We must therefore observe our dreams, pay closest attention and study ourselves just as carefully as we do the patient. Otherwise the entire treatment may go off the rails.[5]

> The doctor who does not know from his own experience the numinosity of the archetypes will scarcely be able to escape their negative effect when he encounters them in practise.[6]

Perry adds that this task of personal and clinical introspection is essential if the therapist is to avoid, "The dangers of blind spots ... and ... the hazards of mutual infection and contagion [by psychic contents]."[7] Looking more at the positive side of this process, psychotherapist and author John Wellwood comments that:

> It is essential for therapists and health professionals to know more about the nature of well-being from within, as it lives inside themselves, in order to better recognize and help awaken it in their clients and patients.[8]

For those who work as carers but are not practicing psychotherapists or psychoanalysts, what are the implications of this? To be more conscious in our caring may mean that we become more effective as healers and less likely to do damage to ourselves or to others in the process. Some basic ideas from psychoanalysis and depth psychology on the psychodynamics of the therapeutic relationship are helpful here.

UNDERSTANDING THE PSYCHODYNAMICS OF CONTAINMENT

Bion's theory of "container/contained" rests on certain assumptions. Foremost among these is that psychological content of the infant

---

[5] Jung (1983), pp. 154-156.
[6] *Ibid.*, p. 166.
[7] Perry (1997), p. 157.
[8] John Wellwood, *Awakening the Heart* (Boston: New Science Library, 1983), p. 57.

(patient), the so-called "contained," can be transferred onto and into the mother (therapist), "the container." There is also an assumption that the mother/therapist/container can then recognize this psychological content of the infant/patient for what it is (i.e., the contained), and hold it until such time as the infant can in turn take it back again. Implicit in this is a further assumption that the mother/therapist is able to contain. These assumptions are based on two of the most widely accepted concepts in psychodynamic thinking, those of *transference* and *countertransference*. As Perry puts it:

> Into the empty space that initially exists between the two parties there emerge the phenomena of transference and counter-transference, an inextricably linked field of interaction that encompasses two people, two psyches; a field of interaction that becomes a major focus of the therapeutic endeavour.[9]

Transference

Psychoanalyst Charles Ryecroft defines transference as:

> 1. The process by which a patient displaces onto his analyst feelings, ideas, etc., which derive from previous figures in his life; by which he relates to his analyst as though he were some former object in his life; by which he projects on to his analyst object-representations acquired by earlier introjections; by which he endows the analyst with the significance of another, usually prior object. 2. The state of mind produced by 1 in the patient. 3. Loosely, the patient's emotional attitude towards his analyst.[10]

These definitions include two further overlapping and related concepts, *projection* and *projective identification*. Projection, which literally means "throwing in front of oneself," is defined as:

> The process by which specific impulses, wishes, aspects of the self, or internal objects are imagined to be located in some object external to oneself. Projection of aspects of oneself is preceded by denial, i.e., one denies that one feels such and such an emotion, has such and such a wish, but asserts that someone else does.[11]

---

[9] Perry (1997), p. 142.
[10] Charles Ryecroft, *A Critical Dictionary of Psychoanalysis* (London: Penguin, 1983), p. 168.
[11] *Ibid.*, pp. 125-126.

Projective identification is defined as:

> The process by which a person imagines himself to be inside some object external to himself. This ... is a defence since it creates the illusion of control over the object and enables the subject to deny his powerlessness over it and to gain vicarious satisfaction from its activities.[12]

Although these definitions are drawn from psychoanalytic theorists, Jung agreed with Freud on the importance of transference. His descriptions of the clinical encounter as an alchemical process highlight the fact that the psychodynamics of relationship are of relevance for *both* the patient *and* the therapist:

> For two personalities to meet is like mixing two different chemical substances: if there is any combination at all, both are transformed. In any effective psychological treatment the doctor is bound to influence the patient; but this influence can only take place if the patient has a reciprocal influence on the doctor.[13]

Jung's views on transference are summarized by Perry as five basic tenets:

1. *Transference is a fact of life:* "In reality it is a perfectly natural phenomenon that can happen [to the doctor] just as it can happen to the teacher, the clergyman, the general practitioner, and—last but not least—the husband." [C. G. Jung, *Collected Works,* 16, para. 358, fn. 16].

2. *Transference needs to be differentiated from the "real" relationship between the patient and the analyst:* ... This aspect of the relationship has come to be known as the "therapeutic alliance," an alliance made between the conscious, adult parts of both parties principally in the service of the patient's developing field of consciousness and expansion of conscious choice through the analytic process.

3. *Transference is a form of projection:* [Jung describes transference as] "A specific form of the more general process of projection ... a general psychological mechanism that carries over subjective contents of any

---

[12] *Ibid.*, pp. 67-68.
[13] Jung (1966–70), 16, "Problems of Modern Psychotherapy," para. 163.

kind into the object ... is never a voluntary act ... is of an emotional and compulsory nature ... forms a link, a sort of dynamic relationship between the subject and the object." [C. G. Jung., *Collected Works,* 18, paras 312-317]. ... An interesting feature of Jung's definition is the phrase "into the object." Projection elsewhere in his writing is thought of as a process of throwing something *onto* someone or something else, just as a projector throws an image onto a blank screen. This definition seems to foreshadow ... Klein's notion of projective identification. ... Within the transference, any aspect of the patient can be projected onto or into the analyst. ... Feelings, ideas, impulses, needs, phantasies, and images are all subject to this involuntary act. ... As the analytic relationship grows and deepens, patients become less concerned with themselves and more preoccupied with the Self. This takes place as the result of working on the personal transference and the withdrawal of projections, of affects, impulses, and other psychic contents that the patient needs for unashamed living.

4.   *Transference has an archetypal [impersonal, objective, universal] as well as a personal [infantile] dimension:* Once these personal contents have been re-owned, Jung noted that,

>   "The personal relationship to me seems to have ceased; the picture shows an impersonal natural process," [C. G. Jung, *Collected Works,* 9, 1, para. 531]. "It goes without saying that the projection of these impersonal images onto the analyst has to be withdrawn. But you merely dissolve the *act* of projection; you should not and cannot dissolve its contents. ... The fact that they are impersonal contents is just the reason for projecting them; one feels they do not belong to one's subjective mind, they must be located somewhere outside one's own ego, and, for lack of a suitable form, a human object is made their receptacle" [C. G. Jung, *Collected Works,* 18, para. 369].

5.   *Transference is in the service of individuation beyond the therapeutic encounter:* Jung attacks the exclusive use of reductive analysis [and of transference as purely an ego-survival/defense mechanism] and suggests the addition of a teleological point of view. The transference is goal-seeking, the goal being the withdrawal of projections by both parties, particularly the patient. ... By 1926, in *Two Essays on Analytical Psychology (Collected Works,* 7), Jung was exploring the question of what happens to psychic energy when it is freed from the personal transference. He concluded that it reappeared as a

"Transpersonal control point ... I cannot call it anything else—a *guiding function* and step by step gathered to itself all the former personal overvaluations." [C. G. Jung, *Collected Works*, 7, para. 216]. This is a clear statement that he saw transference as a dynamic with its own in-built propulsion toward individuation.[14]

Countertransference

Ryecroft defines countertransference as:

> 1. The analyst's transference on his patient. In this, the correct [classical] sense, countertransference is a disturbing, distorting element in treatment. 2. By extension, the analyst's emotional attitude towards his patient, including his response to specific items of the patient's behaviour. ... The analyst can use this latter kind of countertransference as clinical evidence i.e., he can assume that his own emotional response is based on a correct interpretation of the patient's true intentions or meaning.[15]

Countertransference, therefore, describes two processes, which may occur in the analyst in reaction to the patient's transference. The first of these is where the therapist (unconsciously) projects his or her own psychic contents back onto or into the client. This was the classical understanding of the term and was seen as an anti-therapeutic hazard of the analytic encounter. Jungian analyst Michael Fordham calls this *illusory* countertransference and describes it as a neurotic process in the analyst when unconscious conflicts from the analyst's past have been activated, are projected onto the patient and interfere with the therapeutic space.[16] This is the kind of countertransference that Freud told analysts to master,[17] that is, overcome.

The second meaning of countertransference is as a description of the process which occurs within the analyst's psyche as a consequence of the patient's transference. While acknowledging that there are also dangers here, analysts from many and varied backgrounds agree that there is also a very real therapeutic potential if we can recognize and work with this

---

[14] Perry (1997), pp. 142-147.

[15] Ryecroft (1983), p. 25.

[16] Michael Fordham, "Countertransference," in *Explorations into the Self* (London, UK: Academic Press, 1985), p. 150.

[17] Cited in David Sedgwick, *The Wounded Healer: Countertransference from a Jungian Perspective* (London, UK: Routledge, 1994), p. 2.

situation. Fordham calls this form of countertransference *syntonic*. Here, he argues, the therapist is empathetically closely tuned into the patient's inner world and therefore may feel what the patient is feeling, experience what the person is experiencing, possibly even before the patient is conscious of such in him- or herself.[18]

Psychoanalyst Heinrich Racker[19] further subdivides the analyst's own (Fordham's "syntonic") countertransference experience into two types. The first of these he calls *concordant identification,* which describes an empathic sharing of emotional experience. This is where the analyst feels what the patient is feeling; for example sad when the patient is sad, fearful when the patient is fearful. The second he calls *complementary identification.* This notion derives from the theory of projective identification and refers to the analyst's experience as a result of identification with the transferred object of the patient. Here the analyst experiences the emotion(s) the patient is unconsciously split off from and has put into the transference object (as well as his or her own emotional reaction to this material), while the patient's conscious emotional experience at that time is devoid of that or those particular emotions. An example of this is where the analyst may feel sad, angry, and fearful while listening to a patient who has successfully split off these feelings and is describing how serene and accepting he or she feels at this time.

Jung also emphasized the importance of the countertransference:

> You can exert no influence if you are not susceptible to influence. … The patient influences [the analyst] unconsciously. … One of the best known symptoms of this kind is the countertransference evoked by the transference.[20]

> For psychotherapy to be effective a close rapport is needed, so close that the doctor cannot shut his eyes to the heights and depths of human suffering. The rapport consists, after all, in a constant comparison and mutual comprehension, in the dialectical confrontation of two opposing psychic realities. If for some reason these mutual impressions do not impinge on each other, the psychotherapeutic process remains ineffective, and no change is produced. Unless both doctor and patient become a problem to each other, no solution is found.[21]

---

[18] Fordham (1985), p. 150.
[19] Heinrich Racker, "The meanings of countertransference," *Psychoanalytic Quarterly* 26 (1957): 303-357.
[20] Jung (1966–70), 16, "Problems of Modern Psychotherapy," para. 163.
[21] Jung (1983), p. 166.

What is crucial, therefore, according to Jung, is how the therapist responds to this countertransference material. Jungian analyst Harriet Machtiger puts it even more forcefully: "It is the analyst's reaction in the countertransference that is the essential therapeutic factor in the analysis."[22] Commenting on this, Perry adds:

> What she [Machtiger] means here is that the analyst must interpret and make use of his or her subjective responses and fantasies in making sense of the analysand's material and experiences. The skill and competence of the analyst in using this countertransference will determine, in large part, the success or failure of the analysis.[23]

Archetypal Aspects of Transference and Countertransference

Jung stressed that the therapist should also be aware of the archetypal dimension of the transference/countertransference dynamic:

> The transference[/countertransference] phenomenon is without doubt one of the most important syndromes in the process of individuation; its wealth of meanings goes far beyond mere personal likes and dislikes. By virtue of its collective contents and symbols it transcends the individual personality.[24]

In the following quotation Jung identifies the specific archetype which he believes is active within the transference/countertransference dynamic:

> No analysis is capable of banishing all unconsciousness forever. The analyst must go on learning endlessly, and never forget that each new case brings new problems to light and thus gives rise to unconscious assumptions that have never before been constellated. We could say, without too much exaggeration, that a good half of every treatment that probes at all deeply consists in the doctor's examining himself, for only what he can put right in himself can he hope to put right in the patient. It is no loss, either, if he feels that the patient is hitting him, or even scoring off him: it is his own hurt that gives the measure of his power to heal. This, and nothing else, is the meaning of the Greek myth of the wounded physician.[25]

---

[22] H. G. Machtiger, "Countertransference/transference," in *Jungian Analysis*, ed. M. Stein (London, UK: Shambhala, 1985), p. 90.

[23] Perry (1997), p. 158.

[24] Jung (1966–70), 16, "The Psychology of Transference," para. 539.

[25] Jung (1966–70), 16, "Fundamental Questions of Psychotherapy," para. 239.

Jungian psychiatrist Adolf Guggenbühl-Craig explores the relevance of this archetype within the caring relationship.[26] He begins by defining the term "archetype":

> An archetype may be defined as an inborn potentiality of behaviour. Human beings react archetypally to someone or something when faced with a typical, constantly recurring situation. A mother or father reacts archetypally to a son or daughter, a man reacts archetypally to a woman etc. In this sense certain archetypes have two poles, so to speak. The basic situation of the archetype contains a polarity. ... Perhaps we should not speak of a mother archetype, a child archetype or a father archetype. It might be better to speak of a mother–child or father–child archetype.[27]

He proceeds to suggest that this notion of the bipolar archetype is relevant to the process of healing:

> There is no special [single] healer archetype or patient archetype. The healer and the patient are two aspects of the same [archetype]. When a person becomes sick, the healer-patient archetype is constellated. The sick man seeks an external healer, but at the same time the intra-psychic healer is activated. We often refer to this intra-psychic healer in the ill as the "healing factor." ... The physician within the patient himself and its healing action is as great as that of the doctor who appears on the scene externally. Neither wounds nor diseases can heal without the curative action of the inner healer.
>
> ... Many ailments require the ministrations of an external physician. But no physician can be effective without the inner doctor. A physician can stitch up a wound, but something in the patient's body and psyche must help if an ailment is to be overcome.[28]

If the "inner healer" is the pole of the archetype that the patient needs to make contact with, what of the physician?

> Here we encounter the archetype of the "wounded-healer." Chiron, the centaur who taught Aesculapius the healing arts, himself had incurable wounds. ... Psychologically this means not only that the patient has a physician within himself but also that there is a patient within the doctor.[29]

---

[26] Guggenbühl-Craig (1971), pp. 89-101.

[27] *Ibid.*, pp. 89-90.

[28] *Ibid.*, pp. 90-91.

[29] *Ibid.*, p. 91.

Guggenbühl-Craig suggests that because the ego dislikes ambivalence, a splitting of this archetype occurs in the situation of illness leading to a repression of one pole of the archetype and the projection of that pole onto the other. In terms of the transference/ countertransference, this means that the patient represses the inner physician pole of the wounded healer archetype, projecting it onto the outer physician, while the physician represses the inner patient pole of the archetype and projects this onto the patient. Although this may bring some short-term benefits, if the archetype remains split it will soon prove counterproductive:

> In the long run it means that the psychic process is blocked. In such a situation the patient ... may no longer be concerned with his own cure. The doctor, the nurses, the hospital will heal him. The patient no longer has responsibility. Consciously and unconsciously he begins to rely completely on the doctor to bring about improvement. He hands his own healing over to the doctor and, so to speak, sits back and takes it easy ...
>
> In the doctor the repression of one pole of the archetype leads to the reverse situation. He begins to have the impression that weakness, illness and wounds have nothing to do with him. He feels himself to be the strong healer; the only wounds are those of the patients, while he himself is secure against them; the poor creatures known as patients live in a world completely different from his own. He develops into a physician without wounds and can no longer constellate the healing factor in his patients. He becomes only-a-doctor and his patients are only-patients. It is no longer the wounded-healer who confronts the ill and constellates their inner healing factor. The situation becomes crystal clear: On the one hand there is the doctor, healthy and strong, and on the other hand the patient, sick and weak.[30]

But how can this situation be prevented or, if it has occurred, what can be done about it? Guggenbühl-Craig agrees with Jung, Bion, and others who suggest that the onus here is on the doctor him or herself to do the necessary psychological work. How this might be embodied in clinical practice may not, however, be immediately obvious:

> Here we should clarify a possible point of misunderstanding. When I speak of the wounded healer I do not mean a doctor who identifies with the individual patient. That would be pure

---

[30] *Ibid.*, p. 93.

sentimentality and would constitute only an external reunification of the poles of the archetype. Such an identification is a sign of ego weakness, an hysterical method of uniting the opposites.

The image of the wounded healer symbolises an acute and painful awareness of sickness as the counterpane to the physician's health, a lasting and hurtful certainty of the degeneration of his own body and mind. This sort of experience makes of the doctor the patient's brother rather than his master.[31]

Here the doctor has learnt humility and he or she and the patient wait together "close to the ground" for the healing of suffering that is beyond either of their initiative. In this he or she is close to the physicians of ancient Greece, who "maintained that only the divine healer can help while the human doctor merely can facilitate the process."[32] Guggenbühl-Craig concludes by saying:

The doctor can only work creatively if he bears in mind that, despite all his knowledge and technique, in the final analysis he must always strive to constellate the healing factor in the patient. Without this he can accomplish nothing. And he can only truly activate this healing factor if he bears sickness as an existential possibility within himself.[33]

Reflecting on Guggenbühl-Craig's hypothesis, another Jungian analyst, C. Jess Groesbeck, asks the important question, "How [can both] doctor and patient get in touch with their complementary unconscious roles, so that projections fall away, and the "inner healer" of the patient can be activated?"[34] He proposes, "That out of the transference is constellated a "third or higher quantity," that is central to the healing process."[35] This is, he says, "The myth of Asklepios ... reflected in our day in the doctor-patient relationship as an archetypal aspect of the transference."[36]

In agreement with Guggenbühl-Craig, Groesbeck suggests that if this archetypal healing factor is to be experienced by the patient, the doctor must lead the way:

---

[31] *Ibid.*, pp. 96-97.

[32] *Ibid.*, p. 96.

[33] *Ibid.*, pp. 100-101.

[34] C. Jess Groesbeck, "The Archetypal Image of the Wounded Healer," *Journal of Analytical Psychology* 20 (1975): 129.

[35] *Ibid.*, p. 131.

[36] *Ibid.*, p. 127.

If the patient is to experience fully this archetypal image in a dynamic way, the analyst must show him the way. And this can happen only if the analyst first has the courage to experience these powerful archetypal contents. ... [This happens when] the analyst "takes on" the patient's illness or wounds [empathy], and also begins to experience more fully the wounded aspect of the archetypal image. This in turn activates his own wounds or vulnerability to illness on a personal level [countertransference] and/or its connection with the wounded-healer archetypal image.[37]

Only when the doctor has confronted this depth of woundedness in him- or herself is he or she:

ready to re-experience dynamically the healer aspect of the archetype and in this way the phenomenon of wholeness or cure may become effective. If an analyst avoids this painful process he cannot truly be said to be a "wounded healer."[38]

But how much of the patient's suffering should the doctor take on and are there dangers as well as potential benefits in the process?

The question of how deeply involved the analyst should become in taking upon himself the illness of the patient does not admit of an easy answer. While he must get close enough to be involved, activated and aware of his own wounds to catalyse the process [as described], he must also be aware of the dangers of inflation as well as his limitations, including the possibility of his own death and demise. It is precisely the archetypal image of the wounded healer that can help him here. If one "leaves the healing to God," he is much better off. In fact it was God who brought the illness, and hence knows the cure. Hence, though one must be involved deeply, paradoxically, one must not be overzealous in trying to cure.[39]

The penultimate stage in Groesbeck's description of the healing process, from and following on from and only possible because of the doctor's doing his or her own inner work, is when the patient begins to experience healing within him- or herself:

The patient "takes on" the healing strengths of the analyst and also begins to experience the "healer" contents of the archetypal image. This in turn activates his own personal powers of healing and strengths.[40]

---

[37] *Ibid.*, p. 132.
[38] *Ibid.*, p. 133.
[39] *Ibid.*, p. 134.
[40] *Ibid.*, p. 136.

This, Groesbeck says, leads into the final stage in the sequence where:

> The doctor remains as a "healer who is wounded"; the archetypal image of the "wounded healer" remains as before, and the patient, has a "wound healed." At termination, analyst and patient go their way [each] with a portion of divinity within.[41]

He concludes:

> It is only when the healer himself can stay in touch with and experience his own wounds and illnesses as well as confront the powerful images from the unconscious of an archetypal nature, that in turn the patient can go through the same process. For if, indeed, true healing occurs, it would appear that, at least in one form, the wounded physician himself must accomplish it; but the analyst must assist.[42]

Recognizing Countertransference

Countertransference is primarily an unconscious process. How then can the carer recognize that this is what is happening, let alone work with it in a constructive way?

Countertransference may be recognized by the quality and intensity of the feelings it arouses in the carer. Nurse Joy Fest Bonnivier writes, "Countertransference issues have a certain quality of intensity of feeling that distinguishes them from other feelings within a relationship."[43] Patricia Schroder, also a nurse, adds:

> When the feelings are proportional to what is going on, are appropriate to the situation, and are conscious, then it is not countertransference. In contrast ... countertransference should be assumed when strong emotional reactions are experienced that differ from the usual.[44]

Another way of recognizing countertransference is by becoming aware of specific patterns of behaviour it may induce. Writing of this phenomenon in a palliative care setting, Peter Speck says:

---

[41] *Ibid.*, p. 141.

[42] *Ibid.*, p. 144.

[43] Joy Fest Bonnivier, "A Peer Supervision Group: Put Countertransference to Work," *Journal of Psychosocial Nursing* 30 (5) (1992): 5-8.

[44] Patricia J. Schroder, "Recognising Transference and Counter-transference," *Journal of Psychosocial Nursing* 23 (2) (1985): 21-26.

Identification, the consequent loss of boundaries and the difficulty of managing oneself in role in the face of death can lead the professional to develop strategies to minimize the possibility of this happening—conscious and unconscious defences against the emotional impact of the work.[45]

He then describes a number of these defensive behaviour patterns:

Avoidance: Some people ... may avoid the difficulty of talking about death in a personal way by rationalization (the patient doesn't want to know . . .); or by intellectualization (talking in terms of statistics); or by hit and run tactics (telling the patient bluntly and then leaving, avoiding all further contact). Others try to avoid direct contact with death altogether.

Task-centredness and aggressive treatment approaches: The tendency to defend oneself by adopting a task-centred approach is not new. The priest can hide behind the ritual of prayers and sacraments, avoiding interpersonal contact; the doctor can use a stethoscope to silence the questioning patient. ... For clinicians, another way is to move into aggressive treatment approaches with techniques which may prove beneficial in some cases. ... Such a disease-focused approach may be accompanied by a distancing from the patient as a person, and any patient who dies represents a failure. Meanwhile, the human caring aspect is [split off and] vested in the nurse or other paramedic who remains close to the patient and is associated with all that is good, loving and nice. When the patient dies, the nurse may become the recipient of the doctor's negative feelings because of the unaddressed rivalry that has developed between them.

The development of chronic niceness: [Here] ... the individual and the organization collude to split off and deny the negative aspects of caring daily for the dying. There is a collective fantasy that the staff [carers] are nice people, who are caring for nice dying people, who are going to have a nice death in a nice place. This protects everyone from facing the fact that the relationship between the carers and the dying can often arouse very primitive and powerful feelings [countertransference] which are disturbingly not-nice. ... In order that everyone can continue to be nice to each other, the not-so-nice feelings get split off and displaced outside the staff group. For example, there may be much complaining about managers who "don't understand the pressures." ... Similarly, the split-off negative

---

[45] Peter Speck, "Working with Dying People," in *The Unconscious at Work: Individual and Organisational Stress in the Human Services,* ed. Anton Obholzer and Vega Zagier Roberts (London, UK: Routledge, 1994), pp. 95-96.

feelings may be projected on to the patient's relatives [and sometimes the patients themselves], who are then perceived as hypercritical of the standard of care and of the way in which the staff are looking after the patient.

The development of survivor guilt: [The experience that it is others and not us that are suffering and dying can bring about the feeling] ... which psychoanalysts refer to as "manic triumph" ... [and this often] brings with it a sense of guilt (Freud). It can be difficult to acknowledge to oneself, let alone to others, that one feels pleasure in knowing that it is not one's own death or the death of someone important to oneself that is about to happen. In the face of the obvious distress of those who *are* experiencing death, one may then also experience guilt for having survived. There may be a strong desire to split off from and deny such painful feelings.[46]

Speck concludes by describing the sort of measures which may be helpful here:

Such situations cry out for consultation to the staff group and/or management so that these feelings may be contained rather than acted out and projected ... staff groups need space to understand what they are carrying psychologically as a result of the work they do. It is the ability to tolerate ambivalence that can restore integration and the capacity to think. ... The recognition that one can perhaps be *a good-enough* carer for dying people and their families, can be very liberating.[47]

A familiarity with the ideas of transference/countertransference is essential to the therapeutic use of self and the process of containment. So is the ability to recognize and work with the psychodynamics of caring within a clinical setting. As Speck suggests, this is greatly facilitated if carers have the opportunity to reflect on their work in the context of appropriate clinical supervision at a team and individual level.

---

[46] Speck (1994), pp. 96-99.
[47] *Ibid.*, p. 100.

CHAPTER SEVEN

Working with Nature

I feel it with my body,
with my blood.
Feeling all these trees,
all this country
When this wind blow you can feel it.
Same for the country . . .
You feel it.
You can look, but feeling …
that make you.

Feeling make you,
Out there in open space.
He coming through your body.
Look while he blow and feel with your
body . . .
Earth . . .
Like your father or brother or mother,
because you born from earth.
You got to come back to earth.
When you dead . . .
you'll come back to earth.
Maybe a little time yet …
then you'll come back to earth.
That's your bone,
your blood.
It's in this earth,
same as for tree.

Tree . . .
he watching you.
You look at tree,
he listen to you.
He got no finger,
he can't speak.
But that leaf . . .
he pumping, growing,
growing in the night.
While you sleeping
you dream something.
Tree and grass same thing.
They grow with your body,
with your feeling.

Water is your blood.
Water . . .
you can't go without water.

Those trees . . .
they grow and grow.
Every night they grow.
When you cut that tree,
it pump life away,
all the same as blood in my arm

> Well you feel it in your body.
> You say
> "that tree same as me."
>
> This piece of ground he grow you.
> —BILL NEIDJIE[1]

Those who care for others in pain and suffering will have witnessed many moments when "the miraculous" that is healing has happened. They will agree that this moment of healing could not have been prescribed, or willed, or given. When, and if, the healing came, it did so spontaneously, generously and often, surprisingly. It happened within the containment of care. It arose from within the depths of the experience of suffering. It brought feelings of relief, of mutuality, a mix of joy and sadness and a sense of being held in a significance that defied comprehension. We have already considered this process in the mythological terms of Asklepian epiphany and Eleusinian rebirth and we have examined some of the steps we can take to build, with the patient, the secure space where this may happen. What, if anything more, can be done to facilitate this process?

To help answer this question, I would like to introduce another metaphor at this stage, one which builds on much of the imagery already encountered. That is to consider healing as the work of nature within us. By "nature" I am referring to that in our body and psyche that is kindred to the natural realm; to the earth and the trees, to the animals and the rivers.

Finding Our Place

North American poet Mary Oliver writes about kinship with nature. By considering a selection of her writing, we can share in her vision of the natural world as an animated place of healing.

Each morning before dawn, Oliver leaves her house and steps out into what she calls:

> The arena of *things*, the theatre of the *imagination*, the everywhere of *faith*.[2]

---

[1] Bill Neidjie, Stephen Davis and Allan Fox, *Australia's Kakadu Man: Bill Neidjie* (Darwin, Australia: Resource Managers, 1986), pp. 51-61.
[2] Mary Oliver, *Winter Hours* (Boston: Houghton Mifflin, 1999), p. 79.

She goes walkabout in the dreamtime of nature as dawn brightens through the trees, and she brings her attention to whatever unfolds. This is her work and the inspiration for her writing. Her descriptions of outer nature are also a rich portrait of the inner world of soul and spirit:

Landscape

Isn't it plain the sheets of moss, except that
they have no tongues, could lecture
all day if they wanted about

spiritual patience? Isn't it clear
the black oaks along the path are standing
as though they were the most fragile of flowers?

Every morning I walk like this around
the pond, thinking: if the doors of my heart
ever close, I am as good as dead.
Every morning, so far, I'm alive. And now
the crows break off from the rest of the darkness
and burst up into the sky—as though

all night they had thought of what they would like
their lives to be, and imagined
their strong, thick wings.[3]

As Oliver walks through the forest and by the lake, she does so with her eyes and "the doors of [her] heart" open. Her meetings with other beings in this early morning landscape are both ordinary and extraordinary:

December

Then the deer stepped from the woods. It walked from the shadows under the trees into a clear space. Antlers sprang from its brow, each with five or six tines. From the antlers, from each tine, green leaves were growing, as if from the branches of a tree.

The deer stood without moving, brutish and graceful as deer alive in daylight, except that its heavy, elaborate head was carrying, upon the usual curvature of horn, these branches, this fountain of leaves.

Then it turned and vanished. In shyness, perhaps. Or simply because we get no more than such dreamy chances to look

---

[3] Mary Oliver, *Dream Work* (New York: Atlantic Monthly Press, 1986), p. 68.

upon the real world. The door opens a crack, a hint of the
truth is given—so bright it is almost a death, a joy we can't
bear—and then it is gone.[4]

For Oliver the gateway into the natural world is the quality of our
attention. The "attention" she writes about is a focused receptivity of body,
mind, and soul:

> *Have You Ever Tried to Enter the Long Black Branches* (extract)
>
> Who can open the door who does not reach for the latch?
> Who can travel the miles who does not put one foot
> in front of the other, all attentive to what presents itself
> continually?
> Who will behold the inner chamber who has not observed
> with admiration, even with rapture, the outer stone?
>
> Well, there is time left—
> fields everywhere invite you into them.
>
> And who will care, who will chide you if you wander away
> from wherever you are, to look for your soul?
>
> Quickly, then, get up, put on your coat, leave your desk!
>
> To put one's foot into the door of the grass, which is
> the mystery, which is death as well as life, and
> not be afraid![5]

> *The Moths* (extract)
>
> If you notice anything,
> it leads you to notice
> more
> and more.[6]

One possible consequence of attending to nature in this way is that,
in time, we may find ourselves being attended to by nature:

> *Five a.m. in the Pinewoods*
>
> I'd seen
> their hoofprints in the deep
> needles and knew
> they ended the long night

---

[4] Mary Oliver, *White Pine* (Orlando: Harcourt Brace & Company, 1994), p. 51.
[5] Mary Oliver, *West Wind* (Boston: Houghton Mifflin, 1997), pp. 61-62.
[6] Oliver (1986), p. 77.

under the pines, walking
like two mute
and beautiful women toward
the deeper woods, so I

got up in the dark and
went there. They came
slowly down the hill
and looked at me sitting under

the blue trees, shyly
they stepped
Finally
one of them—I swear it!—

would have come to my arms.
But the other
stamped sharp hoof in the
pine needles like
the tap of sanity,
and they went off together through
the trees. When I woke
I was alone,

I was thinking:
so this is how you swim inward,
so this is how you flow outward,
so this is how you pray.[7]

A similar encounter some years later reminded Oliver of this event. Her thoughts in the poem that follows reveal just how significant that earlier meeting was. It had been an initiation, which had moved her from a position of interested observation to one of active participation and interaction:

The Pinewoods

This morning
two deer
in the pinewoods,
in the five a.m. mist,

in a silky agitation,
went leaping
down into the shadows
of the bog

---

[7] Mary Oliver, *New and Selected Poems* (Boston: Beacon Press, 1992), pp. 83-84.

and together
across the bog
and up the hill
and into the dense trees—

but once,
years ago,
in some kind of rapturous mistake,
the deer did not run away

but walked toward me
and touched my hands—
and I have been, ever since,
separated from my old, comfortable life

of experience and deduction—
I have been, ever since,
exalted—
and even now,

though I miss the world
I would not go back—
I would not be anywhere else
but stalled in the happiness

of the miracle—
every morning
I stroll out into the fields,
I believe in everything—

I believe in anything—
even if the deer are wild again
I am still standing under the dark trees,
they are still walking toward me.[8]

From such experience, Oliver speaks of her sense of profound familiarity with the natural world:

> I put my face close to the lily, where it stands just above the grass, and give it a good greeting from the stem of my heart. We live, I am sure of this, in the same country, in the same household, and our burning comes from the same lamp. We are all wild, valorous, amazing.[9]

To know one's kin, to find one's place in the natural world, in what Oliver calls, "the family of things," is to know healing:

---

[8] Oliver (1994), pp. 13-14.
[9] Mary Oliver, *Blue Pastures* (Boston: Beacon Press, 1995), p. 93.

Wild Geese

You do not have to be good.
You do not have to walk on your knees
for a hundred miles through the desert, repenting.
You only have to let the soft animal of your body
love what it loves.
Tell me about despair, yours, and I will tell you mine.
Meanwhile the world goes on.
Meanwhile the sun and the clear pebbles of the rain
are moving across the landscapes,
over the prairies and the deep trees,
the mountains and the rivers.
Meanwhile the wild geese, high in the clean blue air,
are heading home again.
Whoever you are, no matter how lonely,
the world offers itself to your imagination,
calls to you like the wild geese, harsh and exciting—
over and over announcing your place
in the family of things.[10]

In the final pages of her book *Winter Hours* Oliver writes with some
nostalgia and much gratitude of how she feels known and recognized by
nature, and recalls some of the beings and memorable encounters that
have brought her into this awareness:

> Through these woods I have walked thousands of times. For many
> years I felt more at home here than anywhere else, including my
> own house. Stepping out into the world, into the grass, onto the
> path, was always a kind of relief. I was not escaping anything. I
> was returning to the arena of delight. I was stepping across some
> border. I don't mean just that the world changed the other side of
> the border, but that I did too. Eventually I began to appreciate—
> I don't say this lightly—that the great black oaks knew me. I don't
> mean they knew me as myself and not another—that kind of
> individualism was not in the air—but that they recognized and
> responded to my presence, and to my mood. They began to offer,
> or I began to feel them offer, their serene greeting. It was like a
> quick change of temperature, a warm and comfortable flush, faint
> yet palpable, as I walked toward them and beneath their outflowing
> branches.
>
> In the pinewoods is where the owl floats, and where the white egret
> paces, in summer, like a winged snake, in the flashing shallows.

---

[10] Oliver (1986), p. 14.

Here is where two deer approached me one morning, in an unforgettable sweetness, their faces like light brown flowers, their eyes kindred and full of curiosity. The mouth of one of them, and its vibrant tongue, touched my hand. This is where the coyotes appeared, one season, and followed me, bold beyond belief, and nimble—lean ferocities just held in check. This is where, once, I heard suddenly a powerful beating of wings, a feisty rhythm, a pomp of sound, within it a thrust then a slight uptake. The wings of angels might sound so, who are after all not mild but militant, and cross the skies on important missions. Then, just above the trees, their feet trailing and their eyes blazing, two swans flew by.[11]

NATURE AS HEALER

Those in whom we witness healing are those in whom nature has been allowed to do her work. We may remove the obstacles and create the right conditions but the ultimate move is not ours. In her own time and in her own way, nature brings the healing.

If this is the case, how can we as carers best work with nature to help another find healing? We have already considered how the initial moves are to create the containment of care and to understand and work with the dynamics of the therapeutic relationship. We have also seen how this includes the carer's knowing from his or her own inner quest what it means to wait in suffering, and how this itself may bring the one who suffers towards healing, for as psychoanalyst Lionel Corbett puts it:

Personal suffering has a hollowing effect; it allows us the internal space to be able to contain the suffering of others also.[12]

These moves must be accompanied by the carer's turning inwards and downwards towards what Madhava Ashish called "the level from which the healing flows." Finding one's way and learning how to be in this place of nature deep within oneself is a lifetime's work and unique for each person. That we recognize its value and are committed to the search are what seems to be what matters.

If these are the initial moves, are there other ways of working with nature that may help the one who suffers find healing? Jung suggests that there are and indicates where we might usefully focus out attention when he writes:

---

[11] Oliver (1999), pp. 96-97.

[12] Lionel Corbett, *The Religious Function of the Psyche* (London, UK: Routledge, 1996), p. 181.

> Dreams are impartial, spontaneous products of the unconscious psyche, outside the control of the will. *They are pure nature;* they show us the unvarnished, natural truth, and are therefore fitted, as nothing else is, to give us back an attitude that accords with our basic human nature when our consciousness has strayed too far from its foundations and run into an impasse.[13]

> In the dream, the psyche speaks in images, and gives expression to instincts, which derive from the most primitive levels of nature. Therefore, through the assimilation of unconscious contents, the momentary life of consciousness can once more be brought into harmony with the law of nature from which it all too easily departs, and the patient can be led back to the natural law of his own being.[14]

Jungian analyst and author Marie-Louise von Franz echoes this point and hints that dreams may be an expression of an autonomous dynamic towards healing within the psyche:

> As is generally known, we cannot manipulate dreams: they are, as it were, the voice of nature within us. They show us therefore the manner in which *nature, through dreams, prepares us for death.*[15]

If this theory is correct, to work with dreams is to work with nature. And to encourage patients who suffer to attend and listen to their dreams is to help them turn towards a deep, inner, natural source of healing and to allow themselves be carried in its flow.

Although I will be looking at dreams in their literal sense in the remainder of this section, I suggest that we might also consider dreams as metaphor. In this way, "dreams" can be seen as a creative expression of the uncharted wilderness in the depths of psyche. Images are native to this place and so approaches which work with images, such as dreamwork, imagework, art therapy and music therapy, are all ways of working with nature that can be of particular value. Approaches such as body work, meditation, and creative ways of being in actual nature and wilderness can also be considered. Context is crucial here; what matters is that these approaches are practiced within the containment of care, that the carer is committed to his or her own inner process and that they are seen as ways of enabling what is deepest and most natural within the other to unfold and do its work.

---

[13] Jung (1966–70), 10, "The Meaning of Psychology for Modern Man," para. 317.

[14] Jung (1966–70), 16, "The Practice of Psychotherapy," para. 351.

[15] Marie Louise von Franz, *On Dreams and Death; A Jungian Interpretation* (Boston: Shambhala, 1987), p. vii.

CHAPTER EIGHT

Dreamwork as Earth Ascending[1]

The dream is a little hidden door in the innermost and most secret recesses of the soul, opening into that cosmic night which was psyche long before there was any ego-consciousness, and which will remain psyche no matter how far our ego-consciousness extends. For all ego-consciousness is isolated; because it separates and discriminates, it knows only particulars, and it sees only those that can be related to the ego. Its essence is limitation, even though it reaches the further nebulae among the stars. All consciousness separates; but in dreams we put on the likeness of that more universal, truer, more eternal man dwelling in the darkness of primordial night. There he is still the whole, and the whole is in him, indistinguishable from nature and bare of all egohood. ... It is from these all-uniting depths that the dream arises ...

—CARL JUNG[2]

Dreams are the voice of our instinctive animal nature or ultimately the voice of cosmic matter in us. This is a very daring hypothesis, but I'll venture to say that the collective unconscious and organic atomic matter are probably two aspects of the same thing. So the

---

[1] Jay Ramsey, ed., *Earth Ascending; An Anthology of Living Poetry* (Devon, UK: Stride, 1997).

[2] Jung (1966–70), 10, "The Meaning of Psychology for Modern Man," para. 304.

dreams are ultimately the voice of cosmic matter. ... The dream
takes us into the mysteries of nature strange to our rational mind.
                                    —MARIE-LOUISE VON FRANZ [3]

As we wander even further into the materialist desert that our
civilization has become, our dreams are the only oases of spiritual
vitality left to us. They represent our primordial habitat, our last
wilderness, and we must protect them with as much fervour as the
rain forests, the ozone layer, the elephant, and the whale.
                                    —ANTHONY STEVENS[4]

D reamwork, which is taken here to mean attending to and
       being animated by a dream, was central to the ancient rite
       of Asklepian healing. In my experience, dreamwork can be
an especially valuable way of working with patients in suffering, whose
situation closely mirrors that of the Asklepian pilgrim. I agree with the
following words of von Franz and believe that what she says is relevant
to all who suffer: "The voice of nature or the voice of instinct, which is
the dream, helps people to die in peace. It comforts them."[5]

Psychotherapist Janet Muff describes succinctly the value of working
with dreams in people approaching death:

> Although working with thoughts and feelings can be helpful in
> many situations, it may not be enough when someone faces serious,
> life-altering events and the questions they raise. It may be even
> "less enough" when someone faces death. At such times, people
> often find that reason and the problem-solving activities of waking
> consciousness offer few answers and little comfort. In contrast,
> many believe that dreams approach the question of mortality—
> indeed, all the major questions of life—from a much different
> perspective.[6]

The most important aspect of dreamwork is one's attitude to the
image. For the incubants in the Asklepian a dream was nothing less than
an epiphany, a numinous encounter with the god of healing. The first
step in dreamwork, therefore, is to value the dream in and of itself before

---

[3] Marie Louise von Franz and Fraser Boa, *The Way of the Dream* (Boston: Shambhala, 1994), p. 217.

[4] Anthony Stevens, *The Two Million-year-old Self* (New York: Fromm International, 1997), p. 123.

[5] von Franz and Boa (1994), p. 215.

[6] Janet Muff, "From the Wings of Night: Dream Work with People Who Have Acquired Immunodeficiency Syndrome," *Holistic Nurse Practitioner* 10(4) (1996): 70.

attempting any interpretation of it. In this view we appreciate the dream for what it is and, simultaneously, notice therein the web of interconnecting threads which lead in many different directions. One thread leads upwards to that individual's ordinary life with its unique relationships and objective concerns. Another leads inwards to "the personal unconscious" of the individual's subjective experience of emotion and memory. Yet another leads downwards to that in human experience which is shared and universal, where what Jung calls "archetypal" patterns of energy form "the collective unconscious," and beneath that again to what depth psychologist Stephen Aizenstat calls "the world unconscious." This is the level where all is connected in a living matrix:

> The world unconscious is a deeper and wider dimension of the psyche than that of the personal and collective unconscious. In the realm of the world unconscious, all creatures and things of the world are understood as interrelated and interconnected.[7]

From within this context "dream interpretation" takes on a new meaning. It is no longer a move "from above down," so to speak, as we peer downwards into the dark and murky depths with the spotlight of reason. Such an approach reduces dreamwork to yet another cognitive skill and blocks the healing potential of the image. Rather it means allowing rational and objective reality to be interpenetrated by the dream "from below up." As we attend to the dream, as we give it space and allow it to be, it reaches upwards as well as inwards and downwards. This *interpenetration* by the image brings with it a subjective sense of meaning, and healing, and illuminates relevant aspects of our everyday lives.

WORKING WITH DREAMS

The approach to dreamwork outlined here is strongly influenced by the thinking of Carl Jung, James Hillman, and Stephen Aizenstat on imagery and dreams and has evolved within the clinical context of far advanced and incurable illness. Before considering a methodology for working with dreams, I shall firstly consider relevant aspects of Jungian theory, and examine Hillman's phenomenological approach to image and Aizenstat's notion of the world unconscious.

---

[7] Stephen Aizenstat (1995) Jungian psychology and the world unconscious, in *Ecopsychology: Restoring the Earth, Healing the Mind,* ed. T. Roszak, M. E. Gomes, and A.D. Kanner. Sierra Club Books, San Francisco, pp. 95–6.

Jungian Theory

Images are the Primary Language of the Psyche

According to Jung: "The psyche consists essentially of images"[8]; "A psychic entity can be a conscious content, that is it can be represented, only if it has the quality of an image"[9];

> I am indeed convinced that creative imagination is the only primordial phenomenon accessible to us, the real Ground of the psyche, the only immediate reality.[10]

Dreams are, therefore, the primary and native language of the unconscious. They are, Jung says: "A spontaneous self-portrayal, in symbolic form, of the actual situation in the unconscious."[11]

> In each of us there is another whom we do not know. He speaks to us in dreams and tells us how differently he sees us from how we see ourselves. When, therefore, we find ourselves in a difficult situation to which there is no solution, he can sometimes kindle a light that radically alters our attitude—the very attitude that led us into the situation.[12]

Commenting on how and why dreams speak in images, Jung writes:

> It is characteristic that a dream never expresses itself in a logically abstract way, but always in the language of parable or simile. This peculiarity is also a characteristic feature of primitive languages. … Just as the body bears traces of its phylogenic development, so also does the human mind. Hence there is nothing surprising about the possibility that the figurative language of dreams is a survival from an archaic mode of thought.[13]

Jung believed that by attending to our dreams we were attending to the language of our original and deepest nature, our aboriginal self, a source of profound wisdom and healing:

> Together the patient and I address ourselves to the two million-year-old man that is in all of us. In the last analysis, most of our

---

[8] Jung (1966–70), 8, "Spirit and Life," para. 618.

[9] *Ibid.*, para. 608.

[10] Cited in Paul Kugler, "Psychic Imaging: A Bridge Between Subject and Object," in *The Cambridge Companion to Jung*, p. 79.

[11] Jung (1966–70), 8, "General Aspects of Dream Psychology," para. 505.

[12] Jung (1966–70), 10, "The Meaning of Psychology for Modern Man," para. 325.

[13] Ibid., 8, General Aspects of Dream Psychology, paras. 474–5.

difficulties come from losing contact with our instincts, with the age-old forgotten wisdom stored up in us. And where do we make contact with this old man in us? In our dreams.[14]

Jung called the image and symbol-making capacity of the psyche the *transcendent function*. This is described by Jungian analyst Jane Hollister Wheelwright in the following way:

> A pivotal, symbol-forming function, comprising elements of both the conscious and unconscious areas of the psyche. The transcendent function mediates between the conscious and unconscious and transforms their relationship from one of destructive opposition to that of constructive reciprocity and synthesis. Activated by a psychological impasse arising from conflict between opposing attitudes or demands of conscious and unconscious—extroversion/introversion, thinking/feeling, sensation/intuition, masculinity/femininity, spirituality/sensuality, individual/collective—the transcendent function constellates a uniting symbol which synthesizes and transcends the opposites. When assimilated into consciousness, the symbol reveals new possibilities of release from the deadlock and renewal of energy.[15]

The Psyche is a Self-regulatory Dynamic System

Jung viewed the psyche as "A self-regulatory dynamic system based on the flow of energy between opposites";[16] a psychological-ecosystem of sorts, with an inner drive towards homeostasis and balance.

Within this context, Jung saw unconscious contents (such as dreams, fantasies, projections, mental blocks, memory lapses, inappropriate reactions, involuntary behaviour, unexpected thoughts, feelings, wishes and impulses) *as compensatory* in their function:

> Every process that goes too far immediately and inevitably calls forth compensations, and without these there would be neither a normal metabolism nor a normal psyche. In this sense we can take the theory of compensation as a basic law of psychic behaviour. Too little on one side results in too much on the other.[17]

---

[14] Carl G. Jung, *Psychological Reflections; A New Anthology of his Writings,* sel. and ed. by Jolande Jacobi, (London, UK: Routledge & Kegan Paul, 1971), p. 76.

[15] Wheelwright (1981), pp. 285-286.

[16] *Ibid.*, p. 284.

[17] Jung (1966–70), 16, "The Practical Use of Dream Analysis," para. 330.

Although this compensatory or balancing function of the psyche, usually mediated through dreams, is ultimately in the service of psychological integration and growth, this does not mean that it will be experienced as either an easy or pleasant process:

> The more one-sided his conscious attitude is, and the further it deviates from the optimum, the greater becomes the possibility that vivid dreams with a strongly contrasting but purposive content will appear as an expression of the self-regulation of the psyche.[18]

Nightmares can be understood within this framework as dreams, "Whose purpose would appear to be to disintegrate, destroy, demolish. They fulfil their compensatory task in a necessarily unpleasant manner."[19]

The Ultimate Goal of Psychological Work is Individuation

Jung saw psychological work as having both short-term and long-term goals. The short-term goal was to help that individual process and cope with challenges arising from their particular life circumstances. The long-term goal was the achievement of the state of psychological wholeness which he called *individuation.* Jungian analyst Andrew Samuels describes *the individuation process* in the following way:

> A movement towards wholeness by means of an integration of conscious and unconscious parts of the personality ... resulting in differentiation from general conscious attitudes and from the collective unconscious.[20]

Jane Hollister Wheelwright adds the following pertinent comment:

> Jung regarded individuation as a task belonging primarily to the second half of life and as essentially a preparation for death in the sense of growing to perceive and approach death as a normal, integral completion of life.[21]

---

[18] Jung (1966–70), 8, "General Aspects of Dream Psychology," para. 488.

[19] A. Samuels, B. Shorter and F. Plaut, *A Critical Dictionary of Jungian Analysis* (London, UK: Routledge & Kegan Paul, 1986), p. 49.

[20] Andrew Samuels, *Jung and the Post-Jungians* (London, UK: Routledge & Kegan Paul, 1985), p. 102.

[21] Wheelwright (1981), p. 282.

The Individuation Process is Catalyzed by Approaching Death

Approaching death (also understood here in its metaphorical sense as any crisis involving suffering, loss, and a transition into unknown areas of experience) appears to accelerate the individuation process. Jungian analyst and author Edward Edinger comments on this phenomenon in discussing the dreams of a young man he had worked with shortly before the young man died:

> This dream series demonstrates, I think, that the unconscious under certain circumstances brings up considerations which properly can be called metaphysical. Although the dreamer did not undergo the process of individuation in the usual sense of that term, it can be surmised that the pressure of impending death may have telescoped the process. Certainly these dreams suggest an urgency on the part of the unconscious to convey awareness of a metaphysical reality, as if such an awareness were important to have before one's physical death.[22]

Archetypal Activity Plays a Central Role in the Individuation Process

Writing of archetypes, Jung says:

> The collective unconscious, being the repository of man's experience and at the same time the prior condition of this experience, is an image of the world that has taken aeons to form. In this image certain features, the archetypes or dominants, have crystallised out in the course of time. They are the ruling powers, the gods, images of the dominant laws and principles, and of typical, regularly occurring events in the soul's cycle of experience.[23]

> We must constantly bear in mind that what we mean by "archetype" is in itself irrepresentable, but has effects which make visualizations of it possible, namely, the archetypal images and ideas. We meet with a similar situation in physics: there the smallest particles are themselves irrepresentable but have effects from the nature of which we can build up a model.[24]

Polly Young-Eisendrath and Terence Dawson offer the following simple definition:

> [An archetype is] an innate tendency to form emotionally powerful images that express the relational primacy of human life.[25]

---

[22] Edward Edinger, *Ego and Archetype* (Boston: Shambhala, 1972), p. 224.
[23] Jung (1966–70), 7, "Two Essays on Analytical Psychology," para. 151.
[24] Jung (1966–70), 8, "On the Nature of the Psyche," para. 420.
[25] Young-Eisendrath and Dawson (1997), p. 315.

Jungian analyst Edward Whitmont describes how archetypal images may be constellated or activated, when:

> Inner or outer events which are particularly stark, threatening or powerful must be faced [and/or] when there is a state of psychic or physical emergency.[26]

Jung explains how this comes about:

> In any situation of panic, whether internal or external, the archetypes intervene and allow man to react in an instinctively adapted way, just as if he had always known the situation: he reacts in a way mankind has always reacted.[27]

Von Franz develops these ideas within the context of suffering and death:

> It looks as if certain basic archetypal structures exist in the depths of the soul which almost regularly come up to the fore during the processes of dying. ... For whenever man is confronted with something mysterious, unknown ... his unconscious produces symbolic, mythical, that is archetypal, models, which appear projected into the void.[28]

One way these archetypal structures are apparent is in the process of dreaming where they may appear as particular dream-motifs:

> The dreams of dying people show a tremendous variety. Generally they contain the same archetypal motifs which comparative ethnology has discovered in its study of death rituals and the beliefs about life after death among the different human populations: that it is a rebirth, that it is a long, long journey into another country, that it is a transformation, that it is a partial destruction out of which something survives. There are many motifs.[29]

Such an encounter with archetype may bring an experience of healing and integration to a suffering or dying patient. As Jung comments:

> An archetype, rich in secret life ... seeks to add itself to our own individual life in order to make it whole.[30]

---

[26] Edward C. Whitmont, *The Symbolic Quest: Basic Concepts of Analytical Psychology* (Princeton: Princeton University Press, 1969), p. 74.

[27] Jung (1966–70), 18, "The Symbolic Life," para. 368.

[28] von Franz (1986), pp. viii-xiii.

[29] von Franz and Boa (1994), p. 214.

[30] Jung (1983), p. 333.

Perhaps this is what Jungian analyst Albert Kreinheder was describing when he wrote the following words, shortly before his own death from cancer:

> There is a way to die. It doesn't matter when you die so much as how you die. Not by what means, but whether or not you are altogether in one piece, psychologically speaking. I remember frequently those words of Kieffer: "The object of healing is not to stay alive. The object of healing is to become more whole. Death is the final healing." . . .

> As death approaches and the ego weakens, the unconscious leaks through and before long we are almost immersed in the divine. God, as Meister Eckhart envisioned Him, is "a great underground river," and as we are gently, gradually borne upon its waters, we are supremely content and fully healed.[31]

A PHENOMENOLOGICAL APPROACH TO IMAGE

Archetypal psychologist James Hillman proposes a phenomenological approach to imagery and dreamwork. In much of his work, and particularly in his book *The Dream and the Underworld,* Hillman argues for a "re-visioning" of dreamwork. He claims that dreams have been colonized by rational, ego-based schools of psychology and in the process have been devalued, betrayed, and destroyed. Modern psychology, to paraphrase Hillman, could be blamed for the twin crimes of imperialism and genocide when it comes to dreams:

> Each morning we repeat western history, slaying our brother, the dream, by killing its images with interpretative concepts that explain the dream to the ego. Ego, over black coffee (a ritual of sympathetic magic), chases the shadows of the night and reinforces his domain.[32]

At the centre of Hillman's thesis is the primacy of psyche and image over ego and intellect. Although he could and has been criticized[33] for committing the very crime he accuses others of, that is, of taking an exclusively one-sided view of dreams and dreaming, I believe his approach redresses a gross imbalance. In the section that follows, I quote a selection of key quotations from James Hillman's writings on dreams and dreamwork.

---

[31] Kreinheder (1991), pp. 108-110.

[32] Hillman (1979), p. 116.

[33] W. A. Shelburne, "A Critique of James Hillman's Approach to the Dream," *Journal of Analytical Psychology* 29 (1984): 39.

On Interpretation

Each time we take a dream up into life, we reinforce her domination. Every translation of a dream into the bread-and-butter issues of "real" flesh and blood is a materialism.[34]

As long as we approach the dream to exploit it for our consciousness, to gain information from it, we are turning its workings into the economics of work. This is capitalism of the ego, now acting as a captain of industry, who by increasing his information flow is at the same time estranging himself both from the source of his raw material (nature) and his worker's (imagination).[35]

We have to set aside what we naturally and usually do: projecting the dream into the future, reducing the dream to the past, extracting from the dream a message. These moves lose the dream in exchange for what we get from it.[36]

In sleep, I am thoroughly immersed in the dream. Only on waking do I reverse this fact and believe the dream is in me. At night the dream has me, but in the morning, I say, I had a dream. A true subjective level of interpretation would have to keep me subjected to the dream.[37]

By dayworld and daylight, I do not mean the daily world. I mean rather the literal view of any world where things seem as they appear, where we have not seen through into their darkness, their deadly nightshade. It is this dayworld style of thinking—literal realities, natural comparisons, contrary opposites, processional steps—that must be set aside in order to pursue the dream into its home territory.[38]

Interpretation turns the dream into its meaning.[39]

A dream, to remain a dream (and not a sign or a message or a prophecy), can therefore have no one interpretation, one meaning, one value.[40]

Myths say we may not use the sword in the underworld; we may only struggle with the shades in close embrace or throw stones.[41]

---

[34] Hillman (1979), p. 69.
[35] *Ibid.*, p. 118.
[36] *Ibid.*, p. 116.
[37] *Ibid.*, p. 98.
[38] *Ibid.*, p. 13.
[39] *Ibid.*, p. 130.
[40] *Ibid.*, p. 126.
[41] *Ibid.*, p. 114.

On Dreamwork as Conservation and Re-education of the Ego

Conservation implies holding on to what is and even assuming that what is is right. This suggests that everything in the dream is right, except the ego. Everything in the dream is doing what it must, following psychic necessity along the wandering course of its purposes, except the ego. The river must be dry, the bridge so high, the tree uprooted, the dog run over, the party conceal a poisoner, the dentist demand complete extraction—only the ego's behaviour comes under suspicion. It tends to do the wrong thing and make the wrong appraisals, because it has just come from somewhere else and cannot see in the dark. Like Hermes with Hercules, we take the dream-ego as an apprentice, learning to familiarise itself with the underworld by learning how to dream and learning how to die.[42]

The ego is archetypally an upperworld phenomenon, strong in its heroic attitudes until, by learning how to dream, it becomes an imaginal ego.

An imaginal ego is at home in the dark, moving among images as one of them. Often there are inklings of this ego in those dreams where we are quite comfortable with the absurdities and horrors that would shock the daylight out of waking consciousness. The imaginal ego realises that the images are not his own and that even his ego-body and ego-feeling and ego-action in a dream belong to the dream-image. So the first move in teaching the ego how to dream is to teach it about itself, that it too is an image.[43]

On an Archetypal Approach to Dreams

We may compare three approaches to dream persons [images]. The first, let us call it Freudian, takes them back to the actuality of the day by means of association or by means of the objective level of interpretation. Other people are essential for understanding dream persons. The second, which we may call Jungian, takes them back to the subject as an expression of the person's complex. My personality is essential for understanding dream persons. The third, archetypal method, takes them back to the underworld of psychic images. They become mythic beings, not mainly by amplifying their mythic parallels but by seeing through to the imaginative persons within the personal masks. Only the persons of the dream are essential for understanding the persons in the dream.[44]

---

[42] *Ibid.*, pp. 116-117.
[43] *Ibid.*, p. 102.
[44] *Ibid.*, pp. 63-64.

Through [archetypal] dreamwork we shift perspective from the heroic basis of consciousness to the poetic basis of consciousness, recognizing that *every reality of whatever sort is first of all a fantasy image of the psyche.* Dreamwork is the interiorization of earth, effort, and ground; it is the first step in giving density, solidity, weight, gravity, seriousness, sensuousness, permanence, and depth to fantasy. We work on dreams not to strengthen the ego but *to make psychic reality,* to make life matter through death, to make soul by coagulating and intensifying the imagination.[45]

Our image theory means that we have nowhere to place the patient except in his images, in the midst of his "material," and both of us must stay in the underworld, forgoing whatever metaphysical aims the dream might be serving: ego development, integration, social interest, individuation.[46]

Although the dream itself is unconcerned with waking-life ... the dreamwork, as a satisfaction of instinct, will have its effect upon waking-life, even if indirectly and without benefit of the connections to life made by ego-counselling based on dreams.[47]

On Animals in Dreams and Images as Animals

We cannot know what they [animals/images] come for until we first start to wonder.[48]

Generally, animal images are interpreted in depth psychology as representatives of the animal, that is, instinctual, bestial, sexual, part of human nature. ... I prefer to consider animals in dreams as Gods, as divine, intelligent, autochthonous powers demanding respect.[49]

To look at them from an underworld perspective means to regard them as carriers of soul, perhaps totem carriers of our own free-soul or death-soul, there to help us see in the dark. To find out who they are and what they are doing in the dream, we must first of all watch the image and pay less attention to our own reactions to it. As from a duck blind or when downwind stalking a deer, our focus is on the image, acute to its appearance, ourselves abashed, eclipsed in that intensity in order to follow the precise movements of its spontaneity. Then we might be able to understand what it means with us in the dream. But no animal means one thing only.[50]

---

[45] *Ibid.,* p. 137.

[46] *Ibid.,* pp. 195-196.

[47] *Ibid.,* p. 122.

[48] James Hillman and Margot McLean, *Dream Animals* (San Francisco: Chronicle Books, 1997), p. 14.

[49] Hillman (1979), p. 147.

[50] *Ibid.,* p. 148.

The animal presents *a familiaris,* a dumb soul-brother at our side, or a soul doctor, who understands psychic laws other than those of the dayworld ego.[51]

The appearance of an animal restores us to Adam. We recover the first man in the cave, tracing out the animal soul on the underground walls of the imagination. Of course, the different animals present styles and shapes of vitality, so one tends to say, "Animals in dreams represent instincts. They stand for our bestiality and primitivity." No, they do not; first, because they are not ours or us; second, because they are not images *of* animals, but images *as* animals. These dream animals show us that the underworld has jaws and paws, opening our awareness to the fact that images are demonic forces. The least we can do for them is to pay them that primordial respect of the caveman drawing in the dark, face to the wall, that respect of Adam, so closely considering them that he could find for each one its name. We need large caves and loving attention. Then they may come and tell us about themselves.[52]

Studying animals, knowing about them, even feeling for them isn't enough. … We have to *imagine* them. Get into them as imaginal beings, into them as images. That's what Adam did: he looked at these images parading by and read their names out of their natures. He was inside the animal. He knew the animals of his imagination. He and they were all in the same dream.[53]

To read an animal, to hear it, requires an aesthetic perception for which psychology has yet to train its senses. It has yet to find modes of observation beyond laboratory language and the humanoid parallels in the reports of fieldwork. Psychology needs … to rediscover the animal eye of the caveman facing the cave wall, that aesthetic perception which responds to the significance and power of the displayed form. This response begins first as propitiation, as appreciation. We feel grateful that the animal is even there, that it lets itself be seen, that it is a power that has come into a dream, and that this visitation is a momentary restoration of Eden.[54]

What does the animal see and hear and smell when it comes upon another animal? What does it recognize? Without the benefit of a bestiary, its text is the living form. The reading of living form, the self-expressive metaphors that animals present, is what is meant by the legends that saints and shamans understand the language of

---

[51] *Ibid.,* p. 150.

[52] *Ibid.,*

[53] Hillman and McLean (1997), p. 9.

[54] *Ibid.,* p. 17.

animals, not in the literal speech of words as much as hearing the
animals as living presences, pregnant with metaphors.[55]

On Dreams as Meaning Us Well

Whatever the nature, there is a loving in dreamwork. We sense
that dreams mean well for us, back us up and urge us on,
understand us more deeply than we understand ourselves, expand
our sensuousness and spirit, continually make up new things to
give us—and this feeling of being loved by the images permeates
the analytical relationship. Let us call it *imaginal love,* a love based
wholly on relationship with images and through images, a love
showing in the imaginative response of the partners to the
imagination in the dreams. Is this Platonic love? It is like the love
of an old man, the usual personal content of love voided by coming
death, yet still intense, playful, and tenderly, carefully close.[56]

Hillman teaches us where and how to begin as we approach a dream.
His words help to re-educate the "heroic-ego" with its tendency to
slaughter and imprison the animals (images) it meets in the underworld,[57]
into an "imaginal-ego" which attends to all it meets there with humility
and respect.

While acknowledging the value of Hillman's views, Jungian analyst
W. A. Shelburne argues that these must be accompanied by an appreciation
of the positive contribution of the ego to psychological health:

The ego does have a special role to play in the psyche's economy.
… Proper ego functioning is central and essential to adapting to
the kind of world man actually encounters. … Moreover, it is only
because an individual is well-grounded in ordinary consciousness
and ego functioning that the access to altered states and non-egoic
levels of the psyche is able to render him any positive benefit.
Positive outcomes of getting access to depths of the
unconsciousness necessitate, then, a strong ego.[58]

In addition to the primary moves of connecting with and staying with
the image, therefore, there is also need for consciousness and discrimination.
Depth psychologist Diane Skafte's words are pertinent here:

The rational self must always be a full and equal student in any
venture into otherworld encounters.[59]

---

[55] Ibid., p. 75.
[56] Hillman (1979), pp. 196-197.
[57] *Ibid.,* p. 110.
[58] Shelburne (1984), pp. 52-54.
[59] Diane Skafte, *Listening to the Oracle* (San Francisco: Harper, 1997), p. 5.

DREAMING AND THE WORLD UNCONSCIOUS

Stephen Aizenstat's description of the world unconscious builds on Jung's theory of the collective unconscious and Hillman's view that it is "By means of the archetypal image, [that] natural phenomena present faces that speak to the imagining soul."[60] While recognizing the personal and collective dimensions of the psyche, Aizenstat argues that we must acknowledge that the unconscious also has an ecological dimension. His hypothesis rests on an assumption that "All creatures and things are animated by psyche."[61] He elaborates:

> Although there are clear differences in orders of complexity, I make the assumption that all the phenomena in the world possess intrinsic unconscious characteristics—subjective inner natures. ... These inner natures of the world's organic and inorganic phenomena make up the world unconscious.[62]

Within this context dream images are seen in a particular light, and have certain characteristics:

> At the dimension of the world unconscious, the inner subjective natures of the world's beings are experienced as dream images in the human psyche ...
>
> [T]he idea that all beings are ensouled, in and of themselves, locates the life spark *in* the entity, outside of personal human psychic ownership. In this wider view the human experience exists in a field of psychic relationships, one among many. Seen through the "eyes" of the world unconscious, the dream image is an independent presence in a broader psychic ecology, a dreamscape where there is room for many beings to "walk around" and be regarded by one another ...
>
> Dreams, the hallowed windows into the depth of the human psyche, now also provide access to the inner life, the soul, of the creatures and things of our world. Working with dreams, the Depth Psychologist helps cultivate the capacity to hear, from the inside, the voices of those species and objects who help shape our experience, provide the source of our imagination—and who are in need of us.[63]

---

[60] James Hillman, *Archetypal Psychology—A Brief Account* (Texas: Spring Publications, 1983), p. 11.

[61] Aizenstat (1995), p. 97.

[62] *Ibid.*, p. 96.

[63] Aizenstat (1995), pp. 96-97.

Aizenstat is not denying in this the significant personal relevance that dream imagery *usually* has for the dreamer, nor its archetypal significance. Rather he is suggesting that, in addition to this, *if we even begin to allow for the possibility that such images arise from the soul of the world,* then they may also be in the dream for their own independent purposes:

> The elephant that appeared in "my" dream had a life of its own; it visited to interact with me as a fellow creature of the "dreamtime"—perhaps to heighten my awareness of the plight of elephants in the world. From the perspective of the world unconscious, the dreamscape is the worldscape.[64]

Healing is also revisioned here as being more than a purely subjective or, indeed, human phenomenon:

> The time has come to move beyond the widely held belief that psychological health is solely a function of individual wholeness and nurturing human relationships. Although this view has obvious therapeutic usefulness, it exists within a framework that perpetuates the separation of person from world and that denies the essential importance of an individual's surroundings. As Depth Psychologists, we must advocate a reimagining of psychopathology that takes into account the other presences in our world.[65]

Mary Oliver's idea of finding "our place in the family of things" finds echo in Aizenstat's description of healing as an integration with the natural realm in psyche and in the world. Finding our place in this deeper and bigger landscape can ease our suffering by recontextualizing it, can bring a sense of meaning, and can link us to potent sources of creative energy:

> Once we are resituated in this wider, ever transforming ecology of nature, we reconnect with the natural resource and the rhythms that live inside us. Realignment with nature's harmonic provides a potent complement to well-considered medical care.[66]

Finally, Aizenstat tells us that it is especially through the process of attending to dreams, both ours and nature's, that this healing harmonic may come about:

> I believe we must also attend to nature's dreaming, for nature is always dreaming, unfolding herself in each moment. We dream

[64] *Ibid.*
[65] *Ibid.*, p. 99.
[66] *Ibid.*, p. 100.

also—each day imagining ourselves into our own inner nature. In the meeting place between natures, a window opens and we are deeply touched. We remember, for a time, our psychic inheritance, an endowment rooted most essentially in the rhythms of nature.[67]

A WAY OF WORKING WITH DREAMS

The following dreamwork approach is offered as one possible way of working with the dreams of patients suffering from far advanced and incurable illness. The hypothesis underlying this way of working with dreams is that if we listen and attend to our patients' dreams, their psyche can and will do the rest. My experience of working with dreams in a palliative care setting validates the observations of von Franz,[68] Edinger,[69] and others that there is an urgency in the unconscious of patients approaching death to bring certain issues, insights, and attitudes to consciousness. Within this context, a mere turning toward the dream by choosing to give it our conscious attention often appears to be enough to let a process, *which is happening already,* flow more freely and more fully. The implication here is not that all healthcare workers should now become psychotherapists but that they should know how to respond to patients who want to talk with them about their dreams, and that they should be aware of this simple way of working with the healing power of nature.

There are certain provisos to working in this way:

- The carer should work in this way only if he or she wants to and feels comfortable and competent to do so.

- Dreamwork should occur only within the *containment of care,* as already outlined, and in particular within a relationship of trust.

- The carer should have a sense of the limits of his or her skills in dreamwork and readily refer on to others who have the necessary expertise when necessary.

- The carer should have undergone a basic training in dreamwork and have ongoing experience of working with his or her own dreams.

---

[67] *Ibid.*
[68] von Franz (1987), p. vii.
[69] Edinger (1972), p. 224.

- The carer should be supervised in this aspect of his or her work by someone experienced in psychotherapy and dreamwork.

The Aims of Dreamwork

- To enable us to better understand our patients and to help them better understand themselves.[70]

- To enable patients to hear their dream by listening to it with them.

- To work with an inner dynamic towards psychological balance and wholeness by helping patients, through attention to dreams, become more in tune with their deeper selves.

- By working with dreams in this way, individuals may connect to sources of inner strength and wisdom and so experience more fully, deeply, and consciously what they are already living.

Indications for Dreamwork

Some of the most likely reasons for considering dreamwork with a patient are:

- As an integrated aspect of the clinical care of patients who are interested.

- When a patient specifically asks to work in this way.

- Where the patient has been having vivid or distressing dreams and has mentioned this to a carer.

- Where the patient is suffering emotionally or physically in a way which the caring team believes may have a psychological or spiritual basis.

The Process of Dreamwork

Assess Whether or Not it is Appropriate to Work in this Way

On each occasion an assessment must be made as to whether it is appropriate to work in this way with this particular patient. There are certain instances where it may be unhelpful or inappropriate to

---

[70] Muff (1996), p. 69.

attempt to do dreamwork; for example where the patient is delirious or paranoid, or where there is extreme fear or anxiety. Patients who are experiencing a flooding of consciousness by unconscious material need approaches that are ego-strengthening and that validate concrete reality, coupled with a respectful attention to the imagery and emotions they are already experiencing. Such patients are in a waking rather than a sleeping dreamtime and need to be responded to as such. Working with patients' imagery in this setting is a specialized area, which has been well described by hospice nurses Maggie Callanan and Patricia Keely. They call these states of altered consciousness in patients approaching death "nearing death awareness" and outline sensitive and creative ways of responding.[71]

Offer a Rationale for this Way of Working to the Patient

This step, and the one that follows, are partly educational, and ensure that the patient is agreeing to work in this way on the basis of "informed consent." They may also anticipate and help to allay some of the ambivalence and resistance that frequently accompanies the early stages of dreamwork. One needs, in other words, to find ways of introducing dreamwork that gain the trust and co-operation of the patient's *usually* frightened and invariably skeptical ego.

In my experience it is often helpful to begin by discussing the cathartic value of dreaming. I occasionally offer an explanation along the following lines:

> There has been a lot going on for you recently. All this is bound to evoke feelings. While you are aware of some of these, it's quite possible that there are other feelings also but these may be buried so deep that you're not even aware of them. These don't do you any good if they stay bottled up. At night they find a way out in your dreams. In other words, your dreams are a sort of "blowing off of emotional steam." The dreams you're having may not be very pleasant, in fact they can be quite frightening, but it's a good thing they are happening. You're probably being helped by this, even if it doesn't feel like it. Dreamwork simply means helping dreams to do their work more effectively by giving them some of our waking time and attention.

One can then proceed to explain how dreamwork may also be of benefit to them in more positive ways. It may be helpful to describe

---

[71] Maggie Callanan and Patricia Keely, *Final Gifts* (New York: Bantham, 1993).

dreams as a "snapshot" of the inner world at that particular time. Dreamwork, then, is a way of allowing patients to get a fuller sense of how they are reacting and responding to their present circumstances, which brings a clearer sense of what it is they need to help them. Finally, it can be pointed out that while at times of crisis we look for help "outside" and from others, there may also be help on the "inside." One may put this in the following way:

> Deep within us there are untapped sources of healing and wisdom.
> Dreams are a simple and natural way of accessing these.

Describe the Practical Procedure Involved in Dreamwork

If the patient says that she or he would like to try this way of working, a time and place can be agreed to meet. This *usually* entails setting a fixed time aside (ideally one hour) in circumstances that will be private and undisturbed. The patient should be reassured of the confidential nature of the work and know that the session itself will involve looking at particular dream(s) of his or her own choosing and discussing any issues that arise from this. Sometimes, however, dreamwork happens in a much more ad hoc fashion, such as at the patient's bedside for ten minutes or so in the middle of a busy ward round. Even though these circumstances are far from ideal, such brief dreamwork can be of value. The patient him- or herself has chosen this opportunity, which may be a sign that the moment is ripe.

Patients should then be encouraged to begin to record their dreams. It can be helpful to keep a dream-journal in which to write whatever dreams, or fragments of dreams, they recall on waking, no matter how scrappy, trivial, or nonsensical these may appear. Some patients find it easier to use a dictaphone. Very weak patients can dictate their dream to someone else to record. I sometimes make the following suggestions:

> Lie quietly on waking and before doing anything be aware if there are any memories of dreams. If so, observe them for a moment, noting the images and the feeling atmosphere of the dream.
>
> When recording the dream, include as much detail as possible, imagine yourself as you were in the dream, and write in the first person and present tense. Afterwards write down any particular memories, thoughts, or feelings that arose as you were recording the dream.

The Dreamwork Session

Take some time at the beginning of the dreamwork session to discuss the rationale of working in this way, as well as logistical details, especially if these have not already been addressed. Remember that the carer's task is to listen and attend to the dream, with the patient, in ways that allow the psyche to do its work. The challenge here is not to solve yet another problem, as in "interpreting the dream," but to find ways of enabling the spontaneous natural process that is the dream to deepen and unfold. The carer's attitude is crucial in this. The following quotations set the tone.

Jung counsels us to approach the dream with an open mind:

> One would do well to treat every dream as though it were a totally unknown object. Look at it from all sides, take it in your hand, carry it about with you, let your imagination play round it ... [72]

> So difficult is it to understand a dream that for a long time I have made it a rule, when someone tells me a dream and asks for my opinion, to say first of all to myself: "I have no idea what this dream means." After that I can begin to examine the dream.[73]

Hillman encourages us to stay with the image in ways that keep it alive:

> "Stick to the image" (cf. Jung, Ch. 16, para. 320) has become a golden rule of archetypal psychology's method, and this because the image is the primary psychological datum.[74]

> For us the golden rule in touching any dream is keeping it alive. Dreamwork is conservation.[75]

Oliver reminds us that, as with nature, so too with dreams:

> To pay attention, this is our endless and proper work.[76]

Aizenstat tells us that, from an ecopsychological perspective, dream images are:

> Real, have imaginal weight and body, and act in dreams on behalf of themselves.[77]

---

[72] Jung (1966–70), 10, "The Meaning of Psychology for Modern Man," para. 320.
[73] Jung (1966–70), 8, "On the Nature of the Psyche," para. 533.
[74] Hillman (1983), p. 9.
[75] Hillman (1979), p. 116.
[76] Oliver (1994), p. 8.
[77] Stephen Aizenstat (1995) op. cit., p. 96.

Finally, natural historian Barry Lopez's comments on how to relate to landscape suggest a way of entering and being with the dream:

> When we enter the landscape to learn something, we are obliged, I think, to pay attention rather than constantly pose questions. To approach the land as we would a person, by opening an intelligent conversation. And to stay in one place, to make of that one, long observation a fully dilated experience. We will always be rewarded if we give the land credit for more than we imagine, and if we imagine it as being more complex even than language. In these ways we begin, I think, to find a home, to sense how to fit a place.[78]

There are three parts to the dreamwork session itself:

Part 1: Opening

The session begins with the carer inviting the patient to tell his or her dream. The patient will often read from a written account or speak the dream from memory. During this initial telling the carer listens to the factual content of the dream and notes the patient's body language as he or she speaks. In addition, the carer should be aware of his or her own emotional or physical reactions on hearing the dream.

The patient is then asked to retell the dream, including any details that came to mind with the initial telling. On this occasion the carer invites the patient to imagine him- or herself back into the dream and to talk it through in the first person, as if it were actually happening. This is facilitated if the patient keeps his or her eyes closed. As the carer listens to the dream story again, he or she notes any intuitions, images, or daydreams that arise in doing so.

At this stage the carer asks the patient what thoughts he or she has about the dream. This interpretative question may begin to bring the dreamwork session to a conclusion, which could mean that the simple process of the patient's telling the dream, and having it listened to by another in this way, was all that was necessary at this time. The carer then moves directly to the third part of the session and towards ending. Alternatively, this question may open up the dreamwork process and gain the co-operation of the patient's ego by reassuring it that the dream will also be attended to in this way. This then leads into the next part of the dreamwork session.

---

[78] Barry Lopez , *The Rediscovery of North America* (New York: Vintage, 1992), pp. 36-37.

Part 2: Working With

The carer now brings attention back to the dream by asking the patient, "Are there images or aspects of the dream story that particularly strike you, or which seem interesting or curious to you?" The patient is encouraged to talk about each such image, one at a time, initially through association, and subsequently through focusing more closely on the image.

The associations to the dream images may be at any of three levels.

- They may be at an *objective* level, where the dream image seems to connect to actual people or events from that person's past or present experience.

- Alternatively, they may be at *a subjective* level, where the patient begins to talk about feelings, thoughts, or memories evoked by the image.

- Finally, the associations may be at an *archetypal* level, where the dream images remind the patient of myth, art, literature, film, or drama.

The carer's role in this process is to ask questions that help the patient to make these associative connections. The carer will be guided in this primarily by the patient's own choice of what details of the dream to look at, but should also be open to whatever feelings, curiosities, intuitions, or images have been awakened in listening. The responses, comments, or questions that come from the carer's psyche in this way should be presented as feedback, which may or may not "fit" or make sense to the patient, rather than as interpretations.

The carer then brings attention to the particularity of certain dream images by asking the patient for as much descriptive detail as possible. Once again, the carer is guided in which images to look at by the patient's choice and by his or her own intuitive promptings. The patient is invited to close his or her eyes in doing this. This close attention to the image allows it to move from background to the foreground, from past to present tense, as it begins to take on life and body of its own and makes its presence felt.

Although these two moves are presented here in a linear way, in practice it is much more fluid than this and more akin to a serpentine dance. Each move in one direction through association is followed by a move in the opposite direction by returning to the image, weaving a web of connectedness, and deepening the experience of the dream.

Part 3: Closing

The aim of this part of the session is to move towards a conclusion in a manner that allows the patient to gain some understanding from the work just done, to re-engage with objective reality, and to consider ways of keeping the dream alive.

Dreamwork often brings a subjective sense of meaning as something felt and known intuitively, rather than cognitively understood. Analyst and author Laurens van der Post puts it this way:

> [An] awareness of the mystery of things acknowledged and revered, though inexpressible and utterly non-rational, is also a vital form of knowing.[79]

In a similar vein Jung writes:

> Lack of conscious understanding does not mean that the dream has no effect at all. Even civilized man can occasionally observe how a dream which he cannot remember can slightly alter his mood for better or worse. Dreams can be "understood" to a certain extent in a subliminal way, and that is mostly how they work.[80]

That said, dreamwork will often give patients additional insight into their current life circumstances. It is again important that the carer does not offer interpretations at this stage, even if these seem evident. The carer's task here is to contain whatever interpretative thoughts he or she may have, while asking questions which allow the patient to make his or her own connections. It may be helpful to ask what thoughts the patient now has about the dream and in what way these have changed with the dreamwork. Additional questions such as, "Does anything in the dream remind you of how you have been feeling in yourself in recent times?" or "When you think about your dream and about what's going on in your life at the moment, do you see any links or feel any resonances?" are also useful.

The carer then asks the patient: "As you leave the dream and consider what's happening in your life at this time, is there anything you feel you need to do, or say, or ask about, arising from this?" This is a "grounding" question, which locates the patient back in objective reality and shifts the focus of attention towards practical matters and logistical concerns.

---

[79] Laurens van der Post, *Jung and the Story of Our Time* (London, UK: Penguin, 1976), p. 63.

[80] Jung (1966–70), 18, "The Language of Dreams," para. 476.

Finally, the patient is encouraged to consider creative ways of maintaining contact with the living images of the dream in the days ahead. This is possible through art or music, either individually or with the art or music therapist. Other possibilities are ritual, or movement, and by keeping a journal record of feelings, thoughts, memories, and any further dreams that arise. The session ends by agreeing when and where to meet again, if this is what the patient would like.

DREAMWORK IN PRACTICE: PATRICIA'S STORY

> I couldn't sleep a wink last night, doctor. I had the most awful nightmare, which woke me a couple of hours after going to sleep and I tossed and turned for the rest of the night. ... I'm exhausted.

I was on rounds with other members of the ward team and had just introduced myself to Patricia, whom I had never met before. She had been admitted to the palliative care unit the previous day for a two-week respite admission. I knew from an earlier discussion that she had widespread metastatic breast cancer and that she had just completed a course of palliative radiotherapy for an impacted pathological fracture of her right hip.

I was also aware that Patricia was sixty-five years old, an actress and a widow. Her husband had died of a heart attack twenty years previously. That same year the eldest of her three sons was killed in a road traffic accident.

Her two other sons, Ronan and Dermot, lived locally and were very supportive of their mother. Ronan, the elder, was about to leave for Canada for two weeks, which was part of the reason for Patricia's respite admission. Up until recently, Dermot, who was separated from his wife, had been living with his mother along with his two teenage daughters and seven-year-old son, Timmy. Since then he and his children had moved into a new home in a nearby town with his new partner.

Apparently Patricia was fully aware of the nature and extent of her illness. However, the admitting doctor described how she had appeared anxious on arrival on the ward the previous afternoon. She had told him that she felt her admission might have been inappropriate given how well she was, and had needed a lot of reassurance as to the short-term nature of her stay.

Patricia looked worried as she spoke. She seemed weak and as she moved in the bed it was obvious that she was in pain. I said that we could get her something to help her sleep more soundly at night, but it might also be helpful if she were to take time to look more closely at her dream and that I would be happy to help her with this, if she would like. We then spoke about the pain she was getting from her hip and agreed on a plan to change to her analgesia and arrange physiotherapy, which would, we hoped, get her back on her feet again and ready for home.

A couple of days later I got word that Patricia would like to meet me. By then she was a lot more comfortable, had begun mobilizing with the physiotherapist, and was reported to be sleeping better and to be more relaxed in herself. We met in a room off the ward where we would not be disturbed. Patricia was dressed and sitting in a wheelchair. She looked sad but well. I began by telling her that we had an hour for this session and outlined to her how we could look at her dream. I explained to her that the type of dreamwork I was proposing was not so much about dream analysis or interpretation but more a question of giving attention and space to the dream, of listening to the dream. I suggested how this could help, not only by allowing a "blowing off emotional steam" but by helping her to become more aware of what was going on deep inside, since dreams were "snapshots of the unconscious." I suggested that dreams might also allow her to access sources of strength and wisdom deep within herself. I emphasized that it was for her to set the pace and that we would proceed only in a way which she was comfortable with. I then encouraged her to tell me about the dream she had had on the night of her admission and to do this in the present tense and first person singular. She closed her eyes and began:

> I'm on the quayside in Dun Laoghaire. A liner, the *Queen Elizabeth 2 (QE2)*, is there. Timmy, my grandson, is on board. I am meant to get on also but I can't find a door on the side of the boat to get in. The liner is enormous. I'm really worried about Timmy and I want to be with him. Somehow I hear that the liner will dock again at Arklow, so I start running there. I run really fast. When I arrive in Arklow, there's no sign of the *Queen Mary*. I wake in a panic.
>
> I closed my eyes again and tried to make a happy ending, but I couldn't.

As Patricia was speaking, I was both listening to her dream and noticing what feelings it was evoking in me. By the time she had finished, I was aware of a mixture of emotions, including fear and sadness. I then invited her to retell her dream, this time filling in any more details (bold) that came to mind. She retold her dream:

"I'm on the quayside in Dun Laoghaire. **It's busy. There are lots of people there but they don't look at me when I address them.** A liner, the *QE2,* is there, tied up alongside the quay. Timmy, my grandson, is on board. I am meant to get on also but I can't find a door on the side of the boat to get in. The liner is enormous. **All I can see when I look up is this enormous black hill. I know there is more above this but I can't see it.** I'm really worried about Timmy and I want to be with him. Somehow I hear that the liner will dock again at Arklow, so I start running there. I run really fast. **I notice my mother is with me. I feel guilty for making her run so fast.** When I arrive in Arklow **I walk over the brow of the hill and look down into this empty bay.** There's no sign **of the liner. I ask the locals, but they just look at me like I'm stupid.** I wake in a panic."

"Patricia, when you reconnect with your dream in this way, what are your feelings?"

"Mainly fear and worry about Timmy building up to that eventual sense of panic. ... There was also a sense of awe towards that enormous liner."

"What about Timmy?"

"Timmy is my youngest grandchild. He's seven but he's very small for his age. When Dermot separated and moved in to live with me, Timmy was three. He's been with me for the past four years. I've been like his mother. He moved into their own house in Bray four weeks ago. Dermot's partner is very nice; she likes the kids and they her. I know I may die from this but I'm so worried about Timmy, even though I know he'll be well cared for. He knows that I'm very ill but not that I'll die."

"I can sense something of how worrying and how sad this must be for you, Patricia. I can see how you have been like a mother to Timmy. It must have been very hard for you to see him moving out—even if you knew he would be loved and cared for."

I was aware as I said this that her fractured hip and hospitalization must have happened very shortly after these events. This would have compounded her experience of loss and led to her transfer to the palliative care unit and a confrontation with another imminent separation, as dark and awesome as the "enormous black hill" on the quayside.

"I noticed your mother appeared by your side on the way to Arklow, the second time you told the dream."

"My mother was on a lot of committees, the ICA [Irish Countrywomen's Association] and so forth. We always seemed to be moving house, my brother and I. She wasn't over-affectionate but she was always there when I needed her. We weren't at all alike."

"Anything in particular about Arklow?"

"I really dislike the place. It's scruffy. The sort of place you pass through. No sense of belonging there."

"What about the *QE2?*"

"I've no idea. ... It's just that Timmy is so young. He's so small and vulnerable. I'm worried about how he's going to manage in the town ... strange people about. At least when he was with me, he was safe. I live in Wicklow at the side of the Sugarloaf [mountain]."

"I noticed that in your first telling of the dream, the *Queen Elizabeth* became the *Queen Mary.*"

"Yes, I was aware of that too as I said it. I've no idea why. I always seem to get the two mixed up."

"If you look at the dream as a whole, do you feel or see any connections when you think about what's been happening for you lately and what you're going through?"

"I came in because my son Ronan was going to Canada. I didn't want to come here. I couldn't sleep that first night and lay there awake and frightened. Whereas last night I also couldn't sleep but I felt relaxed. I wasn't so afraid. ... I'm really worried about Timmy ... I'm glad to know that the social worker is going to get involved and meet with Dermot."

By now the hour was up and we agreed to leave it there. Patricia said she was surprised that the time had gone so quickly. I suggested that we could meet like this again early the following week, if she so wished, and encouraged her to continue to record her dreams in the meantime.

In the days immediately after this session, Patricia had more pain and seemed to be very anxious at times. She had episodes of panicky breathlessness and needed frequent contact and attention from her son Dermot. He had stayed overnight with her in the dayroom on the night before we next met. Patricia was keen to meet with me again and this was arranged. She began the session by telling me of two dreams she had had on the previous two nights:

In the first dream I'm in this hospital setting, surrounded by these people—professionals. I don't recognize them. I'm giving birth. I've given birth to the baby's head but the strange thing is, it doesn't have a face and I don't have a sense of its body—perhaps it's still in the birth canal?

The following night, I seem to be in the same setting and I think the same people are standing around. It feels as though there's a definite link with the previous night's dream, but this time I've given birth to a baby. While I'm not clear about its features, what is clear is that it's a whole baby and it's in my arms and I'm *thrilled.* The strange thing is that there's no reaction from the people around me—none.

Also, I had this dream the second night I was here: I am trying to climb up this enormous wall. It's black, slippery, wet. There are no footholds. It's hard to climb. I'm alone. The higher I climb, the higher the wall gets. Somewhere up there, I can see the sky. Over to the side I can see some workmen. One of them is wearing a red jumper. I'm not sure what they're doing. Maybe they're knocking down this wall, or another one? I shout, "Help me!" They hear me but they just ignore me. I lose my confidence and fall in panic.

I felt somewhat overwhelmed and breathless at this stage. I asked Patricia which of the three dreams she would like to look at. "The wall dream," she replied. As she had been telling me that dream, I had been struck by similarities between it and her boat dream. It seemed as if this latter dream was in many ways a continuation of the first dream. The feelings it had evoked in me were of fear, hopelessness, and panic.

"You describe that black wall so vividly. Does anything come to mind when you think of it?"

"No, although it reminds me a bit of the black wall in front of my house. In fact, I *know* it's to do with that wall, although that wall is much lower. In front of my house is a driveway and a lawn that slopes down to that wall. It's black and slippery and wet on the far side from the river. The river gets really high in the winter. One night when the kids were little, as I turned my car to leave for a rehearsal after supper I pressed the accelerator instead of the brake by mistake and lost control. The car went crashing down the lawn and over the wall and ended up nose down in the river. I went to open the door but I couldn't as both my hands were trapped like this. [She puts her hands together in the praying position.] I remember the engine of the Volkswagen roaring. I thought it might explode. Then my husband noticed the lights flashing and came and rescued me. ... I always meant to do something with that wall. It's so ... menacing."

"The way the workmen ignored you in this dream reminded me of how the people you spoke to in the boat dream also seemed to ignore you. Do you feel any connections here?"

"No ... except while I'm really happy that Dermot has such a wonderful partner ... I also feel a bit redundant now ... ." [It was obviously difficult for her to say this.]

> "The fact that you are delighted that things are working out so well for Dermot and his family doesn't take away from the enormity of the losses you are living at the moment and all the feelings these evoke."

> "Yes, and fracturing my hip at the same time as they moved out meant that I lost my independence at the same time as I lost my role. ... My family are so important to me. We are so enmeshed. Losing my husband and Michael that same year was *huge*. It affected us all and made us very close."

Patricia was also concerned about her continuing tiredness, the fact that she had so little energy and wanted to talk about this.

> "How can I fight this if I haven't even the strength to go out to the loo on my own?"

> "There are different ways of "fighting." The old way meant lots of effort and willpower, but perhaps what's happening these days could be seen as another way. Your dreams show that there's an awful lot going on inside. You're dealing with such change and so much loss and all the feelings this brings up. That's real and important work and it takes lots of energy. It may be that this is where your strength is going. Maybe right now it's not so much about understanding 'why?' so much as allowing that this work is taking place because it needs to take place. Perhaps 'fighting' at the moment means choosing to trust what is happening."

As the session ended, Patricia spoke about how excited she was at the prospect of getting home that coming weekend. Dermot would be there with his children and she was looking forward to seeing her beloved dogs.

I next saw Patricia five days later. The weekend at home had been a great success. The plan was to have another week of intensive physiotherapy in the unit and to be discharged home by the weekend. As I came to her bedside on rounds, Maura, the ward sister, told me that Patricia wanted to speak with me. I was struck by how well Patricia looked. She was obviously animated as she began to speak:

> I wanted to tell you. ... Something fell into place about the big boat as I sat in the car on my way back here last night. When I a little girl my mother died. Because my father couldn't cope I was put into an orphanage. That was in Wales. When I was four I was sent to live with my aunt in Ireland. (This aunt became my "mother.") I remember, so vividly, standing as a little girl with my suitcase on the quayside looking up at this giant boat, heading into a new world ...

Patricia was so excited to have made this link, which she felt was very significant. I felt in awe at her psyche's ability to create the dream and to make such a healing connection. She spoke of how the feelings of being ignored and not being listened to in both dreams also felt related to this early experience. She then turned to me and asked, "What do you see as the value of dreamwork?" I was a bit thrown by the question. I replied:

> Well ... like I said when we met recently, I see dreamwork as a way of paying attention to dreams as expressions of our deepest feelings and thoughts and of an untapped wisdom we each carry within ourselves. It doesn't seem to be primarily about helping us to understand what's going on, although that often happens as well, so much as helping us to see what's happening in a new way and to remember important things. Dreamwork seems to help things fall into place for a person—like pieces of a jigsaw.

A few days later Patricia was discharged, almost two weeks after the day of her admission. She returned home without pain and very much more mobile than she had been, with more energy and in good spirits. I met with her before she left and since she said she was not remembering her dreams, we did not make any definite future appointment.

I next met Patricia about a month later. Following four successful weeks at home, during which time she had been visited by the home care team, she had been readmitted because of a new onset, severe pain in her right arm. Radiographs had revealed partial collapse of a number of vertebrae in her cervical spine due to tumor and this had been treated with a cervical collar, corticosteroids, and urgent radiotherapy. Her pain had settled down and luckily she had not developed any weakness of her arms. One day on my rounds she mentioned to me that she had been dreaming and that she would like to meet me again. We arranged a session for later on that day.

> At home my dreams were joyful, happy dreams and this was true when I first came back in here a couple of weeks ago. This has changed in the last week or so ... they've become very active ... like one I had last night of soldiers' feet marching past; the noise, the activity ... and last Monday night I had a dream I want to tell you:
> I am in one of the houses where I lived as a child (we moved a lot and lived in a lot of old stately homes). I am about twelve in the dream. I'm in the sitting room of this house. It looks like it's hardly used. It's beautiful. I had wanted this as my room with its beautiful furniture and lovely printed material on the couch. ...

Anyway, in the dream, there's a garden right up the centre of the room and it's full of flowers of all colours, reds, yellows ... and you're there and I'm delighted with this and to be able to show it to you. You think it's great. I can just walk past and pick flowers for anywhere in the house. Then smoke, black smoke, starts to come out of the chimney and begins to fill the room. I can't breathe or see easily. It's getting worse. Strangely, there is no sense of danger or pain. Dermot and Ronan are there. They are their present age ... but I feel very embarrassed; it ruins what was there.

I was aware of feelings of wonder at the beauty of the room and its amazing, magical garden, of some surprise at finding myself in the dream, and of alarm at the invasion of this space by the ominous black smoke. I was interested by her comment that there was "no sense of danger or pain."

"When you tell your dream, I get a sense of wonder at this extraordinary garden in the beautiful room. And then the black smoke; making it difficult for you to see or breathe. I was particularly struck by your saying that you had 'no sense of danger or pain.'"

"Well, Ronan and Dermot were with me. They decide for me, they make me feel safe. And the embarrassment; that seems related to how I feel now that I am no longer able to fulfil my role as church organist. I don't want to let them down. When I was started on the steroids a couple of weeks ago, I felt so good, I got on to some of the church choir and suggested that we should begin preparing some choral music for Christmas. I feel so embarrassed to think I may not now be able to go ahead with that."

"How would you feel if you didn't have to do this?"

"Relieved."

"And the smoke, the black smoke that fills the room, does it feel like it's related to anything you've been feeling lately?"

"Yes! I've felt cloudy in my head at times and I'm terrified of this. Am I going mad? Is the cancer moving from my neck to affect my brain?"

"No, Patricia, you're not going mad and cancer doesn't spread like that, from neck to brain. This cloudy, muzzy feeling you describe could be related to some of the medication changes you have had in the last couple of weeks. Also, you've been speaking of how physically exhausted you've been feeling. Well, your brain is part of your body and this 'cloudy' thinking could be a symptom of brain exhaustion."

"No one realizes how tired I am."

Before finishing, we discussed if she would like me to phone her church and let them know that she would not be there to play the organ that coming weekend. She did not want me to do this but later that day asked one of her sons to phone through her apologies.

Over the next couple of weeks Patricia's condition weakened considerably. She appeared to be very comfortable but was intermittently and increasingly confused. We could not find any obvious medical cause for this; her blood tests, including her serum calcium, kidney, and liver function, were normal and there was no improvement even though we reduced or discontinued any sedative medications she was on. There was a possibility of brain secondaries, but this did not seem likely since she was still on high doses of corticosteroids, and did not have any localizing neurological signs or symptoms of increased intracranial pressure. It seemed as if the confusion was part and parcel of her general weakening and not something we could reverse with specific treatments. What was remarkable was how calm Patricia herself seemed to be in her confused state. During my meetings with her at this time, the thought occurred to me that she was now *in* her dreams and that she seemed able to be in them without being overwhelmed or terrified. I spoke to her in these terms and encouraged her to let these thoughts and imaginings be and to allow herself to go with what was happening. Her family and certain members of staff were distressed to see her like this but they seemed to find some comfort in the reassurance that Patricia herself did not appear to be suffering and to know that if she did show signs of distress or agitation, she could immediately be given some tranquillizing medication.

I called in to say goodbye to Patricia on the afternoon of the nineteenth of September as I was going to be away for the next couple of days. She was sleeping peacefully and her daughter-in-law was at her bedside. When I called her name, she briefly opened her eyes and tried to focus on my face. I do not know if she recognized me or not and she immediately sank back into a deep sleep. That evening she developed a high temperature and became somewhat restless. The nurses removed her cardigan and duvet and she settled. Her family, who had been sitting with her, then went home for the night. In the early hours of the following morning Patricia once again became restless and began to call out. Rachel, the nurse on duty, gave her an injection of a tranquillizing medication and called her family since it was evident that she was beginning to die. Patricia's breathing became rapid and once again she started to call out. Rachel repeated the tranquillizing injection and Patricia settled back to sleep. About half an hour later she died, with a friend and Rachel at her bedside. Her sons arrived shortly afterwards.

Review of Patricia's Story

It may not be sufficiently evident from the above account that Patricia's story unfolded within the intricate web of relationships with her devoted family and the multidisciplinary ward team. Patricia had become close to a number of the nurses and her work with the physiotherapist, the art therapist, and the social worker was significant. My relationship with Patricia as her doctor and the dreamwork we did together should be seen, therefore, as just one piece in a bigger pattern of care.

One way of viewing Patricia's story would be to recognize that her suffering, her relationships of trust with those caring for her, and her being in the palliative care unit were all aspects of creating the alchemical *vas bene clausum,* the essential containment of care. Within this, the interdisciplinary care and treatment she received further strengthened the container, while helping to clear and hold an inner subjective space. These various circumstances were also akin to the pilgrim patient's arrival at the Asklepian, the rituals of preparation and the eventual entry into the sacred space of the temple. All that could be done had been done. The task was now to wait in the darkness knowing that the initiative for whatever might happen next was not ours.

The First Session

On hearing Patricia's first dream, I was immediately struck by the immense power of the archetypal image of the giant black boat about to leave the harbor. It reminded me of a scene in Fellini's film *Amarcord* when, out of the silence and hopelessness of the villagers' night watch, an immense liner with all its lights blazing moves by in utter silence. Awe, majesty, wonder, dread; the sorts of feelings one might expect to feel in the presence of the divine. Instead of looking at the numinous quality of the images, however, Patricia chose to focus on Timmy, her beloved grandson, and her feelings of anxiety, panic, and grief at the thought of losing him. This dissonance between the aspects of the dream I wanted Patricia to look at and those aspects of the dream she wanted to look at herself served as a reminder to me that this was *her* dreamwork and not mine, and that my task was to encourage her to go wherever the images led her.

It was difficult for me to witness and sense Patricia's emotional pain as she spoke, through the medium of the dream images, of her imminent death and the feelings of fear and sadness this engendered. I longed to reassure her. "If only she'd look at the archetypal aspects of her dream, it may bring some comfort!" I thought to myself. In practice, I find it *very* hard to sit there as a doctor and allow a patient to be in pain. I feel responsible and find it very difficult to believe that this emotional distress could, in some way, be to that person's benefit. Although this says something about me as a person, it also says something of the difficulties of doing dreamwork as a doctor. A question we must ask ourselves here is: "Whose hat are we wearing when we do dreamwork—Hippocrates's or Asklepios's?" It seems to me that the former is very hard to take off! However, as a supervisor used to say to me, "We have to trust the patient's psyche." Perhaps this is what wearing an Asklepian hat in dreamwork entails: a letting go of the omnipotent fantasy implicit in the Hippocratic approach, while realizing that the healing of suffering happens, when and if it does so, deep within the psyche of the one who suffers, and that this comes about in its own time and in its own way. In the Asklepian mode our task is not "to make it better." It is to help to create the space where the one who suffers is held in trust.

I was aware of the similarity of my feelings on first hearing the dream to Patricia's as she began to discuss it. It is as though a dream is a living tissue embodying a mix of images and emotions and these are transferable to the one who listens to the dream. The question here is what do we do with the countertransference, that is the feelings and thoughts evoked as we listen to the other recounting or discussing his or her dream? I believe that we must begin by being aware that these are *our* feelings and *our* thoughts. Although it may be appropriate to find a way of reflecting back some of the feelings evoked in listening, it is usually inappropriate to offer interpretations at this stage. To do so is to risk killing the process dead as we come in with *our* agenda. Validation of this position seemed to come when Patricia made her own interpretative connections some ten days after the initial dreamwork session. The recognition that her feelings on the quayside in the dream were those she had had as a four-year-old girl heading into the unknown felt hugely important to her. This act of remembering became an act of deep re-membering.

The fact that Patricia was described by the nursing staff as "not good" after the initial dreamwork session, with an increase in pain and anxiety in subsequent days, allows me to re-emphasize an important characteristic about dreamwork. Assuming that at least some of the increase in Patricia's emotional distress following the session was attributable to the dreamwork (it is, of course, possible that it was due to other unrelated events) is a further reminder that dreamwork is not just another Hippocratic intervention. Dreamwork is not a psychotherapeutic equivalent of Valium or morphine. Whereas the aim of an Hippocratic intervention is cure, in the sense of controlling or fixing the problem, the goal of an Asklepian approach such as dreamwork is healing, in the sense of integrating more fully into conscious awareness previously unconscious or alienated aspects of ourselves, which sometimes means confronting "difficult" emotional and psychological material. Enabling a person to become more aware of and in touch with who they are and what they are living, does not mean that this will be either an easy or pleasant experience. The process of healing may be a painful and difficult one, at least in the short term, which creates real challenges for a health care culture that is so completely identified with the Hippocratic values of "pain relief (yours and mine) at all cost and as quickly as possible."

The Second Session

It seemed to me that in many ways Patricia's second dream was a continuation of the first. By reconnecting her with her memory of her terrifying car accident, it appeared to bring her even more deeply into those feelings of blackness and complete helplessness that were also present in her first dream. It was as though her psyche was repeating those particular aspects of the previous night's dream, which she needed to experience more fully; her psyche's own amplification process.

I was heartened by this since it appeared to validate the hypothesis that the psyche is doing its own work anyway. Each night every one of the patients in our care is dreaming, and healing is happening spontaneously, autonomously, independent of and even despite us. What dreamwork means is making this process more conscious, by facilitating and catalyzing what is already happening. As von Franz puts it:

> It is as if nature slowly broods on the problems, developing them slowly. ... Our conscious attention can speed up that maturing process by co-operating with nature in working out problems.

> Analysis is nothing else than the concentration of our conscious
> attention upon that natural maturing process to speed it up. It's
> like adding fire, so that the process will go faster.[81]

In the memory the second dream evoked, Patricia was rescued by her husband. Now, in her present objective circumstances, she once again found herself in the blackness of the unknown, utterly alone and helpless. But who was going to rescue her on this occasion? I for one certainly wanted to and longed to offer my interpretative thoughts and reassurance as a balm for her emotional distress. Were I to have done so, however, I may have acted out the countertransference in an unhelpful way. Although this would have made me feel better and possibly even comforted Patricia in the short term, it might not have been what her psyche needed. More on instinct than insight, I once again chose to hold back. This seemed to create space for her unconscious to act allowing her to make her own associations and connections.

Perhaps I should say at this point that there are also situations where it is entirely appropriate and helpful to share something of our experience as we listen to and respond to what the other is saying. What is then important is *how* we do this. We must be careful to share this material as *my* response to what *you* are saying. For example, we might say something like "When you say that, I get a sense of . . ." or "When you describe that part of your dream, I am reminded of . . .." By qualifying what we are saying in this way we are offering something of ours, which the other may or may not choose to use as they listen to, amplify, and clarify their own experience.

The Third Session

The hyperactive tone to the dream fragments Patricia described at the beginning of the third session ("marching feet," "noise," "activity") may have something to do with the high-dose corticosteroid medication, which she had just been started on. These can cause an acceleration of thought processes, which may be reflected in a person's dreams. That is not to say that the dream content is a mere side-effect of medication. A dream may still contain very relevant imagery even if this is heightened or coloured by medication.

I responded to Patricia's third dream by summarizing some of my feelings on hearing the dream and asking her what aspects of the dream

---

[81] von Franz (1994), pp. 210-211.

she would like to look at. She chose to focus on the black smoke and her reactions to it. There was quite a contrast between how she said she felt in the dream ("no sense of danger or pain") and the tangible fear in her voice as she asked about the clouding of consciousness she had been experiencing of late. What was the psyche's purpose in this dream? In retrospect, the black smoke appears to have been an accurate description of the terminal confusional state Patricia was beginning to experience at that stage. As well as this, there was the image of the beautiful, indoor garden. Was this an image of the Self? And was Patricia's psyche portraying what was happening while giving her what she needed to hold her and carry her through this experience and the days ahead? Indeed, it was striking how calm Patricia actually was in the confusional state, which persisted until her death some two weeks later. Somehow she could be in the confusion without fear, as though she was in a safe place within herself from which to watch the clouds of thoughts and images swirling past.

Overview

Looking back on Patricia's story, it was certainly not a question of the dreamwork "making it all better." As we have seen, she appeared, if anything, more distressed in the immediate aftermath of the first dreamwork session and, although this settled, she experienced further feelings of anxiety, disappointment, and sadness during her final weeks. Although she was mostly well and seemed content during this time, there are many possible reasons (besides dreamwork) for why this might have been so. The "improvement" that was so evident in Patricia within two weeks of her admission to the palliative care unit could be explained by a combination of her own resourcefulness, her family's support, and the Hippocratic interventions and the good palliative care she had received. Against this backdrop we might ask what difference, if any, dreamwork made for Patricia?

My recollection of Patricia is of a beautiful and sensitive person with an enormous love for her family, who gradually seemed able to let go of her concerns and to allow herself be carried with great dignity through her final weeks as both body and mind weakened. During this time she remained interested in all that was happening and very much alive. I believe that the dreamwork she did played a part in enabling her to live her dying in this way.

Patricia used the dreamwork as she wanted to. Her dreams helped her to discuss her concerns about her family, to experience and express an array of deep, powerful, and sometimes painful emotions, and to reconnect with memories, which were hugely significant to her. Meanwhile, the fact that her psyche was also preparing her for death was evident in the archetypal quality of certain dream images—the boat pulling out of the harbor, the newborn baby, and the beautiful room with its flowering garden. It is as though while Patricia was focusing on the surface with all its objective and interpersonal concerns, the deeper layers of her psyche were independently working on another agenda. In parallel to all the outer work, an inner ritual of leave-taking was simultaneously taking place.

When Patricia had asked me what I saw as the potential benefits of dreamwork, I concluded my reply by saying that dreamwork can help "things fall into place for a person, like pieces of a jigsaw." Dreamwork, as part of a bigger picture of care and support, enabled some of the pieces of the jigsaw of Patricia's experience to fall into place. This allowed her to be more herself and to live more completely and consciously. It is also possible that by familiarizing her with her dream images and by educating her into a way of being with them, the dreamwork was a rehearsal of sorts for the altered state of consciousness she experienced in the "confusion" of her final two weeks. Through the dreamwork Patricia found a way of being in the dreamtime of her confusion without so much fear as she might otherwise have had.

I was saddened when I heard that Patricia had appeared distressed and called out just before she died. Whatever else the dreamwork may have done, it appeared not to have protected her from whatever it was she encountered on death's threshold. I felt some guilt about this and questioned the value of this way of working. I tried to rationalize what had happened as being due to her fever, but that somehow did not seem an adequate explanation. Then I remembered how Patricia had told me during the first session about a recurrent nightmare she had had from childhood until a few weeks after her husband's death. In this, an amorphous black shape came towards her and began to envelop her until she awoke screaming. Some weeks after her husband's death she had this dream again, but on that occasion she felt her husband's hand on her arm. "It *was* his hand . . ." she had insisted, "and I didn't move my arm for some time afterwards so it wouldn't go away." Since then she had never had that nightmare. Then I recalled her dream images of the enormous black boat, the black wall, and eventually the blinding, suffocating black smoke. Were these latter-day appearances of the same amorphous black shape of her childhood nightmares and was this what had reappeared shortly before she died? Had we not engaged with the blackness enough to protect her from its return? On the other hand, had the dreamwork at least allowed Patricia to begin to differentiate certain elements of this ominous shadow? And did she feel a reassurance akin to her husband's touch when Rachel comforted her shortly before she died? I do not know the answers to any of these questions. While dreamwork can illuminate some of the inner world of the person in suffering, we must realize that, at best, it is like peering into the vast depths of the ocean. There is so much there we do not or cannot ever see or understand.

SECTION IV

EDUCATION

CHAPTER NINE

Educating the Wounded Healer

As he approached his own death, François Mitterrand, the late President of France, wrote of healing in suffering in the following way:

> At the moment of utter solitude, when the body breaks down on the edge of infinity, a separate time begins to run that cannot be measured in any normal way. In the course of several days, sometimes with the help of another presence that allows despair and pain to declare themselves, the dying take hold of their lives, take possession of them, unlock their truth. … It is as if, at the very culmination, everything managed to come free of the jumble of inner pains and illusions that prevent us from belonging to ourselves.[1]

Perry tells us that, by the end of the therapeutic (analytic) encounter, the experience of wholeness may be shared by patient and carer alike:

> Both patient and analyst have travelled further along the path of individuation; both have been transformed by the work. The patient hopefully has introjected the analyst as a helpful figure, and has internalised the analytic relationship, which will continue to act as a positive, potent inner resource, particularly during difficult

[1] Cited in Marie De Hennezel, *Intimate Death: How the Dying Teach Us to Live* (London, UK: Little, Brown, 1997), p. ix.

times. The analyst likewise has enlarged and deepened his or her clinical experience and expertise, and has changed primarily as a result of his or her mistakes and failings.[2]

Returning to Bion's model of "container/contained," Emmanuel reminds us of the potential rewards of containment, while cautioning that this process also has very real dangers:

> In ... the countertransference, the feelings may be aroused in the therapist for the purposes of communication as described by Bion, i.e., requiring a period of sojourn in the therapist's mind, the container, undergoing transformation through being thought about and then handed back in a more tolerable form to the person. This is helping the person bear something unbearable, making sense for him, the true meaning of containment. ... The therapeutic task and skill lies in choosing the appropriate moment to hand the feeling back. However, if the feeling has not been detoxified enough by being experienced and thought about long enough by the therapist and the therapist attempts to hand it back too soon, the patient will feel that the therapist is just trying to push the feeling back into him and experience it as an assault. The therapist would be felt then as the hostile communication rejecting container and a vicious circle will set in, where the person may try and re-project the feeling again with increasing force. If the therapist can accept the projection of the feeling, i.e., let it in and survive its sojourn in his or her psyche, without totally falling prey to it himself, then the person may again or for the first time develop a belief that a container does exist for [his or her] most primitive feelings.[3]

Just as the healing may be experienced by patient and physician alike, so too, when things go wrong in the process of containment, both parties may suffer. For the patient, the experience of lack of containment and/ or a "faulty container" can result in an amplification of his or her suffering, an increased sense of isolation, and an "acting out" of the distress in behaviour that is self-destructive.[4] For the carer the potential dangers are also real, multiple, and may harm the carer him- or herself and/or the therapeutic relationship. These include the situation of the carer reacting unconsciously to countertransference feelings of dislike, anger, or fear in ways that may be mutually damaging. There is also the risk of what Jung called "unconscious infection" and of the "illness being

---

[2] Perry (1997), pp. 154-155.
[3] Emmanuel (1996), p. 6.
[4] *Ibid.*, p. 4.

transferred to the doctor"; where the carer falls ill (physically or psychologically) because of unconscious contagion by the patient's psychic contents in the transference.[5] Finally, there is the danger of "inflation,"[6] where the carer, unconscious of the splitting of the wounded-healer archetype, overidentifies with the "healer" pole of the archetype and feels and acts like God in a manner that turns his patient into an object of his power drive.[7]

Given the healing potential of relationship and given that there is also the risk of failure and danger here for both patient and carer alike, how can we best prepare ourselves for the challenging task of conscious caring?

In the world of psychoanalysis and depth psychology this takes the form of a training analysis and ongoing clinical supervision. But what might this mean for other workers in healthcare and for the family and friends of those suffering with far-advanced and terminal illness? What might a preparation and education in the essential elements of Asklepian healing—containment, the therapeutic use of self, and the ability to work with the healing power of nature—look like in practice?

CORE CONCEPTS

Recognition of the need for and value of inner/personal work as a central and integral part of healthcare training

Training in the vast majority of healthcare disciplines is predominantly knowledge- and skill-based. Implicit in this is the assumption that what really matters in the healthcare business is how much we know and how skilled we are at putting this into practice. In essence, this is a training which is informed *only* by the values of Hippocratic medicine. While acknowledging the strengths and values of this type of approach, an education in Asklepian healing begins with the recognition that when dealing with suffering, a different emphasis and a different focus is needed. The basic premise in educating the wounded healer is the understanding that who we are as carers matters. The therapeutic use of self calls for a commitment to inner work to run in parallel to the outer work of Hippocratic training.

---

[5] Jung (1966–70), 16, "The Psychology of Transference," para. 365.
[6] Groesbeck (1975), p. 134.
[7] Guggenbühl-Craig (1971), p. 94.

An understanding of and an ability to work with the psychodynamics of the healing encounter

This involves gaining an understanding of issues of transference and countertransference, an ability to recognize countertransference when it occurs and finding ways of working with and dealing with such dynamics in ways that facilitate the healing process.

An appreciation of the archetypal nature of healing

Whereas in Hippocratic medicine the healthcare worker can experience him- or herself as the agent that brings about the cure, in Asklepian healing the ultimate agent of healing is the "divine." This means that the healthcare worker needs to appreciate that, although he or she plays an active role in creating a secure containing space for the patient's suffering, the healing, when, and if, this comes, does so from a realm beyond either party's will or effort. We need to be aware that in caring for another in suffering, the most we can do, as psychotherapist David Findlay puts it, is "to prepare and hold the space where the miraculous may happen."[8]

A familiarity with approaches which enable the patient to open to and access deeper levels of his or her own psyche

For a majority of patients in suffering, inner healing appears to happen spontaneously within the containment of care. Both this group of patients and those whose suffering appears intractable may benefit from approaches such as dreamwork, imagework, art therapy, music therapy, massage, body work, and meditation, all of which can be seen as ways of co-operating with and catalyzing the deep, natural healing potential of the psyche.

METHODOLOGY

The essential knowledge base of Hippocratic medicine can be taught didactically, but Asklepian healing must be learned experientially. There is a knowledge base here also but this should be taught within the context of personal experience.

---

[8] David Findlay, personal communication, 1989.

Inner/personal work

This is the most important component of education in Asklepian healing, building on the premise that who we are as carers is the cornerstone of the healing process. "Physician, know thyself" is where it begins. As we have already considered, this does not mean having it "all sorted out" (psychologically speaking) before being able to attend effectively to our patients. It does mean, however, having an awareness that who we are as persons is the containing space for the one who suffers. Working with personal experience in the clinical setting could happen in a variety of ways. For example, students could be asked to keep a journal recording their feelings and reactions to clinical encounters. The students could then meet with a clinical supervisor experienced in the psychodynamics of caring on a regular basis. Another possibility would be for students to undergo personal psychotherapy, again on an individual or group basis, throughout their training and to continue with personal and clinical supervision at a postgraduate level.

Apprenticeship

This means spending time with others more experienced in the ways of the wounded healer. The most important teachers here are patients themselves, and imaginative ways should be considered to allow students to share in their patients' experiences of illness and suffering. An anthropological approach could be used where, for example, a student is given one or more patients with chronic disability or illness to befriend and follow throughout their training. Another possibility would be for the student to spend time in the home of such a patient and his or her family and participate in that patient's daily care, including attending hospital outpatients and visiting when the patient is in hospital. Apprenticeship may also involve the students spending time with psychotherapists, art and music therapists, and others working primarily from the Asklepian model.

Experiential workshop teaching

Workshop teaching using techniques such as visualization, reflective questioning, and role play, can allow students to experience and reflect on many of the psychodynamics of the healing encounter in a controlled and safe way. The experiential workshop format can also be used to introduce students to ways of recognizing and responding to patients' unconscious communications and to methods of working with the inherent healing dynamic of the psyche.

CHAPTER TEN

Workshops on the Therapeutic Use of Self

I now present an outline of two half-day workshops that have been run for international, mixed-discipline groups of postgraduate students in palliative care over a number of years. They are offered as examples of the type of experiential workshops that can be of value in helping students in health-care to become more aware of the dynamics of the healing encounter and of the phenomenon of the wounded healer.

WHY WORK ON OURSELVES?

Students participating in workshops such as these should be there by choice. If students are there against their will, they may resist or disrupt the work-shop, which will be counterproductive for all involved. Ideally, therefore, the workshops should be publicized in some way beforehand, so that students know the general content and methodology of what is involved and have a choice as to whether or not they attend. Even students who do choose to attend may be suspicious or anxious about participating. As already stated, students in healthcare are, for the most part, unfamiliar with this way of working. Their ambivalence to committing themselves is in part because such an approach is so at odds with the rest of their education programme. It could also be because this way of working poses a threat to their own unconscious defence systems, a hypothesis supported by evidence showing that doctors may have above average fears concerning death and illness.[1] It is, therefore, hardly surprising that some students may at first be less than enthusiastic about participating in such forms of teaching.

On the basis of what I have just said, it is obviously imperative to set a clear context for this way of working at the beginning of such an experiential workshop. This, along with a more detailed description of the methodology and reassurance that students can participate in whatever way feels safe and acceptable to them, allays much of the anticipatory anxiety.

When running these workshops in a palliative care setting, the facilitator might begin by telling students of David Tasma's previously cited words to Cicely Saunders: "I only want what is in your mind and in your heart."[2] This allows the point to be made that while our patients want what we know, they also expect, and need, something of who we are.

The facilitator then discusses Saunders's concept of "total pain,"[3] with which the students may already be familiar. The dynamic entity that is total pain is made up of many different layers or levels or components— for example, the physical, the emotional, the social, and the spiritual— and although most of this pain responds to intervention, not all of it does. Some aspects of total pain, such as grief, do not respond to intervention and call for a different understanding and approach. This "other approach" involves more than our knowledge and skills; once again it demands something of who we are as persons.

Next, the facilitator introduces the concept of suffering as a metaphor for those aspects of the patient's experience of illness that do not respond to intervention. He or she reminds students that people in suffering usually, in their own time and in their own way, find a way of living with and possibly through their suffering. This, combined with the fact that the healing of suffering seems to come from within the person him- or herself, means that our task in this situation is a very different one from

---

[1] H. Fiefel, "Functions of Attitudes Towards Death," in *Death and Dying Attitudes of Patients and Doctors* (New York: Group for the Advancement of Psychiatry, 1965), pp. 632-634.
[2] du Boulay (1984), p. 56.
[3] Saunders (1978), p. 194.

when we are helping a patient in pain. "Helping" a person in suffering means finding ways of enabling that person to endure and live with his or her experience. The best way of doing this is to stay with that individual in his or her suffering. This is not easy, for it also brings us into suffering. Finally, the facilitator makes the point that the more we as carers can be with our own suffering, the more encouraged and enabled our patients are to do the same. Helping our patients in suffering, therefore, has a lot to do with *who we are* as carers.

This initial explanation of rationale is used at the start of either of the following workshops. Occasionally these two workshops are run back to back in the order they are presented below. At other times they are run individually, perhaps as part of a wider course.

Whose Pain is it Anyway?

Before beginning the workshop proper, the facilitator explains the methodology that will be used. This involves some reflective questioning, reflective exercises, writing notes for themselves, working in small groups, and some large group discussion. The facilitator will again acknowledge that for most of the group this may be a very new way of working and may bring up some feelings of anxiety. Having a clear sense of the rationale of the workshop, knowing the methodology to be used, and being reassured that each student can take the workshop at whatever pace and level of involvement feels right for them can create the necessary level of trust and safety that such workshops require. The facilitator(s) may also feel some anxiety at the beginning of such workshops. Again this is understandable, given the fact that, even though they may have run this workshop many times before, each new group has its own unique process and dynamic, which cannot be anticipated beforehand. Careful planning and debriefing afterwards with an experienced supervisor are essential for the facilitators of such workshops.

Part 1

Exercise

The first part of the workshop begins by inviting the students to close their eyes and by leading them through a brief centering exercise, which brings their attention inwards. They are then asked to remember a time when they were with someone in suffering; no matter how hard they or anyone else tried, they could not take that person's suffering away. They remember the person and the details of the circumstances of the encounter, and as they do so, recall how they were *feeling* and how they *reacted* at the time.

The students are then invited to leave this remembered event and come back to the present and, when they are ready, to open their eyes. They next take a few minutes to write notes for themselves in response to the two questions they have considered. When they are ready, they are asked to join up with other students in groups of three or four to share as much of the remembered story as they want to. Their task is to try to identify with the others in the group any common feelings or reactions. After a time for group discussion, the facilitator asks students first for their feelings and then for their reactions, which are written on two separate flip charts.

Teaching

Although each group of students is different and produces new questions and ideas, there are some general themes which repeatedly emerge in doing this workshop.

At the end of this initial exercise, students will have named a wide variety of feelings—for example, fear, panic, helplessness, compassion, the desire to help, confusion, the wish to get "out of there"—which will have been written on a flip chart. The facilitator may then ask the students to consider how the person in suffering might have been feeling and again document their responses. Students are amazed to see the similarity between both lists of feelings. This raises questions about the transmissibility of emotion, and allows for a brief introduction to the ideas of transference and countertransference.

Commonly identified reactions include "trying everything I knew to make it better," "feeling numbed and not knowing what to do," "asking the advice of real experts in the field." The facilitator can then describe the three basic ego-survival reactions of "freeze" (going numb from the neck down), "fight" (doing, doing and doing more), and "flight" (usually by referring the patient on to someone else). Many of the feelings and reactions shared by the students can be understood in this context. The facilitator may also point out the difference between "reaction," which describes an unconscious action triggered by a stimulus, and "response," which describes a conscious choice to act on a stimulus in a particular way. The facilitator emphasizes that there is no one right or wrong way to react and that most reactions in such situations will yield positive and helpful results, not least because they usually come from an underlying desire to help the one who suffers. It needs to be appreciated, however, that not all reactions are helpful. Sometimes they have more to do with protecting ourselves and lessening our own distress and feelings of impotence in the face of the other's suffering ("whose pain is it anyway?") and may not only be counterproductive but positively harmful. The most important fact here is that we each recognize our own individual pattern of reaction in the presence of suffering. This does not stop us reacting in the same way on the next occasion, but it does give us the space to consider whether or not this mode of action is the most appropriate way of responding to this particular situation.

Part 2

Exercise

Once again the students are asked to close their eyes and to bring their attention into themselves. They are then asked to remember a time when they themselves were in suffering. All that could be done had been done but the suffering was still there. They are asked to recall the circumstances of this time and to remember how they felt and what they did to try to ease their distress. They are asked to recall one person whose presence or support helped or made a difference to them at that time. Even though this person could not "fix it" for them, their contact nonetheless made a difference. As they are invited to begin to come back to the present, they are asked to consider the following questions:

- "Do you see any similarities between your feelings and reactions here and the situation where you were with the other person in suffering?"

- "What was it about the person's approach that made a difference to you in your suffering?"

- "How would you describe the quality of this person's approach?"

- "If your experience of suffering was changed by this encounter, in what way was it different?"

The students then write notes for themselves. During the discussion that follows, the facilitator writes the qualities of the person the students remembered on a flip chart and invites their comments and observations.

Teaching

When the facilitator asks if any students saw a similarity between their feelings and reactions in both parts of the exercise, this is often the case. With this may come the realization that our pattern of feeling and reaction to suffering in others is largely determined by how we react to the suffering in our own experience.

When students are asked to describe the approach and qualities of the person they remembered, they frequently use words like "gentle," "humorous," "vulnerable," "respectful," "accepting," "intuitive," "present," "loving," "compassionate," and "wise." What consistently emerges is that it was *who the person* was, rather than anything that he or she said or did, that mattered. That is not to deny the value of that individual's skill and expertise, which on many occasions will be described as having been crucial to the outcome. Even in these instances, however, the students emphasize that it was *how* the person was with them, in particular the experience of not just being listened to but being heard and of being emotionally held in a secure, accepting way that was the crucial factor.

In response to the question of how their experience of suffering differed, if it did, after the encounter with the other person, students often describe this in the following way:

> The ache was still there but it was different to how it had been. Before it was overwhelming; I could think of nothing else, there was room for nothing else. After, I could think of other things also, it felt like there was less pressure ... more space. I could breathe. I could live with it now.

This allows for discussion and teaching on the profound effects that simply being met and heard by another person can have on the experience of suffering. The observation is frequently made that the person in suffering no longer felt so isolated. Although they may speak of having still felt alone in their experience, as a result of the meeting with the other the barrier of isolation was broken and they were better able to live with this sense of existential aloneness, which seems to be an integral characteristic of the human experience of suffering. This distinction between "isolation" and "aloneness" seems important, and students readily understand it.

Conclusion

In the final part of this workshop, the facilitator may refer back to the concept of pain and suffering as metaphor, which will already have been spoken about in the introduction. At this stage, having been through the experience of the exercise, the students may be able to relate to these ideas at an intuitive as well as a cognitive level. This allows teaching, if appropriate, on the need for the two distinct but intertwined models of care to help patients in *both* their pain and their suffering. The person in pain needs the knowledge and skills of the medical model and of evidence-based medicine, which describes what we know and what we do to cure, control, or fix the problem and return the status quo. Additionally, the person in suffering needs what might be called "the wounded healer" model, which recognizes that the secure space (containment) that the person in suffering requires may best be provided by one who is able to be with and allow his or her own experience of suffering.

WHO AM I WHO CARES?

This workshop may be run as a follow-up to the "whose pain is it anyway?" workshop, in that it continues to explore the themes of the inner healer and the nature of the healing encounter. Alternatively, it can be offered on a stand-alone basis.

Introduction

In addition to addressing the question "why work on ourselves?" and discussing the difference between pain and suffering, the students are introduced to the following model around which the workshop exercises are organized:

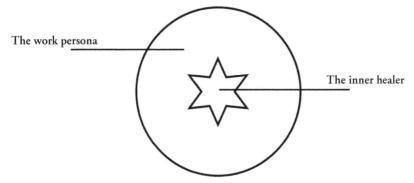

The work persona

The inner healer

"The work persona" describes the outer, visible aspect of our working self, the "white coat" or "uniform" we put on whenever we enter our workplace. This is the part of ourselves that we and others know and recognize as "nurse x" or "doctor y." It has to do with our particular area of professional expertise and competence. "The inner healer" is not so easy to describe. It has to do with the inner, hidden, deeper aspects of ourselves as carers and influences how we do what we do (the quality of our work) and who we are in our work.

Students are told that the workshop is designed to help them get a clearer sense of who they are as carers because this is related to the quality of their work and their ability to help patients in pain and suffering. They are told that there are three parts to the workshop:

- a reflection on the strengths and limitations of their work persona

- an exercise to help get a clearer picture of who or what the inner healer means to each of them

- an examination of how these two parts of themselves as carers work together in a healing encounter with another.

It is hoped that this will allow students to distinguish some of characteristics of such healing encounters and also to get a clearer sense of the role the patient him- or herself plays. Students are told that the methodology will include the use of picture cards as an aid to reflective questioning and are encouraged to pace themselves in a way that feels safe.

Inclusion

As a way of beginning the workshop, students are asked to consider the question:

- "How am I feeling in myself as I begin this workshop?"

They are told that in a neighboring room they will find a selection of photographs and postcards displayed on tables. These cards depict a wide variety of subjects and themes, many of an abstract nature. Staying in touch with the focus-question, they are then asked to go, silently, to the neighboring room and to take their time to consider the picture cards laid out there. When they see an image that seems to "fit" or "speak to" them in terms of their question, they should choose this image and bring it back with them. When everyone has returned, each person introduces themselves and says as much or as little about how they are feeling in terms of their chosen image. This is usually done by going around in a circle.

Part 1. The Work Persona

Exercise

Students are initially taken through a brief centering exercise. They are then asked to picture, in their mind's eye, themselves arriving at their place of work; to notice what they are wearing, the way they move, the expression on their face. They are then asked to see themselves meeting with a colleague and again asked to notice how they interact, their body language, and how their colleague seems to react to them. Finally, they are asked to picture themselves with a patient and once again to notice how they interact and how the patient reacts to them. As they begin to leave this inner place and prepare to return to the here and now, they are asked to consider the following questions:

- "How do you feel towards this work persona you have just been observing?"

- "What do you see as the strengths of this work persona?"

- "What (if any) do you see as its limitations?"

Having written notes in response to these questions, the students are invited to share some of what they have noticed in a small group with two or three of the other students.

Part 2. The Inner Healer

Exercise A

Referring back to the diagram of the work persona and inner healer on the flip chart, the facilitator acknowledges the difficulties in grasping what is meant by the inner healer but emphasizes the importance of attempting to do so if we are to appreciate and work with some of the deepest aspects of ourselves as carers. The facilitator suggests that it may be easier to understand what "the inner healer" means for oneself if one has firstly attempted to recognize how this appears in another. He or she then leads the students through a brief reflective exercise and poses the following questions:

- "Think about someone whom you consider to be a 'healer' in the deepest sense of the term."

- "What, in your opinion, makes this person a healer?"

The facilitator then asks the students to open their eyes and invites answers to the question:

- "Can you name the particular qualities which this person seems to embody?"

The facilitator writes the students' comments on a flip chart.

Exercise B

This exercise helps students to reflect on the significance of the inner healer. Once again they are asked to close their eyes. After a centering exercise, the facilitator leads the students through a guided meditation, which brings them more deeply into themselves. He or she eventually asks them to consider the question:

- "What does the inner healer mean for me?"

While staying in touch with this question, and remaining in silence, the students are once again asked to go into the room where the cards (now either a new set or a much expanded set of those used for the earlier inclusion exercise) are laid out. Music can be played in this room and the lighting arranged in a more muted way to emphasize that this is liminal space and different from the everyday world of the classroom. Once again the instruction is to take time, in silence, and to "allow the image to choose you." They then return to the classroom with their chosen image. At this stage the students are asked to write notes for themselves in response to the following questions:

- "What attracted you to this image?"

- "Describe what you see in this image of the inner healer."

- "What does the inner healer mean for you?"

When the students have had time to do this, and having acknowledged that this exercise may have brought individuals to a place deep within themselves, the facilitator invites any student who wishes to share his or her chosen image with the group, with emphasis on describing the image rather than analysing or explaining it. In the sharing that follows, students are thanked for what they say, but there is no further discussion of their individual contributions at this point.

Part 3. The Healing Encounter

Exercise

After a brief centering exercise, the students are asked to remember an occasion in their work which they would call a "healing encounter." They are asked to take their time to fill in the details of the encounter— the other person involved, the circumstances, and their own role in this. They are asked to recall what were the consequences of this encounter for the other person, for themselves, and for their relationship with the other person. As they leave this memory and begin to come back to the here and now, they are asked to take some time to consider and write notes on the following questions (which are written on the flip chart):

- "Why do you remember this as a healing encounter?"

- "In this encounter, what do you perceive as the role of your work persona?"

- "How did the inner healer come into this encounter?"

- "What was the role of the other person in this encounter?"

- "Can you identify and name the qualities this other person embodied?"

- "What were the consequences of this encounter for the patient, for you, and for your relationship with the patient?"

Large group discussion

Plenty of time (usually an hour or more) is left for this final part of the workshop. The six questions the students have just been considering act as a backdrop to this large group discussion. The diagram of the work persona/inner healer and the qualities of the person they considered a "healer" are also still on view. The facilitator *usually* begins by reading aloud the first question ("Why do you remember this as a healing encounter?") and waiting for one of the group to respond. The teaching is built on issues that emerge as individual students tell the story of the encounter they remembered and in the ensuing discussion of these and the other questions.

The Work Persona

Although one of the principal aims of the workshop is to allow students to get a clearer sense of what is meant by the inner healer and to affirm this potential in themselves, it is essential to firstly acknowledge the positive strengths and values of their work persona while recognizing that this also has its limitations. If it were not for the work persona, the majority of the students would not have been in the situation which became the healing encounter. The work persona, based on the medical model of problem-solving, helps to create the secure environment in which the encounter happens. In addition, the work persona acts as a protection for the carer ("clinical objectivity") allowing him or her to move into and stay close to situations of pain and suffering without getting overwhelmed in the process. At the same time we need to realize that the work persona does not have the ability to "cure suffering" and that to simply relate from this part of oneself as carer to the patient would limit that relationship to what Jewish philosopher Martin Buber describes as an, "I-it" way of relating.[4] This objectification of the other in that relationship can be diminishing for both parties and prevent the deeper dynamics of the healing process from unfolding. Furthermore, an overidentification by the carer with his or her work self (and the inevitable alienation from the inner healer, which follows on from this) can have damaging long-term effects on the quality of the carer's work and lead to carer burnout. An examination of the work persona in the healing encounter shows the value of this aspect of who we are as carers, while demonstrating how it is just one part in the bigger picture of the healing process. We must not become overidentified with our work persona (e.g. "I work as a doctor" rather than "I am a doctor") and learn the art of knowing when and how to step "beyond the white coat" as human beings to be with another in suffering.

---

[4] Martin Buber, *I and Thou*, trans. Walter Kaufman (Edinburgh: T & T Clark, 1970).

The Inner Healer

These aspects of who we are as carers concern what we already know at the level of instinct, intuition, and wisdom; in other words, they have to do with who we are as persons. The inner healer works hand in hand with the work persona, which not only "prepares and holds the space" in which the healing encounter may happen, but also allows the inner healer access to the one who suffers. The inner healer has to do with whatever it is that happens in the hidden depths of the healing encounter. To relate from this place in ourselves to the other in suffering is what Buber calls an "I-thou" way of relating,[5] that is whole person in relationship to whole person. It is important to appreciate that there are also risks in overidentifying with these aspects in oneself. These include the dangers of the carer being overwhelmed by the patient's suffering, and of becoming "inflated"[6] and mistakenly thinking that he or she is the source of the healing.

It is also valuable to discuss how the work persona and the medical model which underpins it is the "dominant culture" within healthcare, while the inner healer and the model of the wounded healer is very much a "minority culture" and as such may be seen as an object of ridicule or threat by the status quo. This allows for some introductory teaching on "terror management theory."[7] Those interested in developing the wounded healer model in their own practice must take this into account and put the necessary supports and protections in place (in particular, adequate training and individual or group supervision).

Another possible topic for discussion at this point is the role of the imagination in healing. For many students the exercise of finding an image of who or what the inner healer means for them feels deeply significant. There is certainly a sense of being in the presence of something numinous or sacred when students share these images in the group at the end of this exercise. Students often speak of the sense of awe their image inspires and may have great difficulty in handing the photo back at the end of the workshop (with frequent requests for photocopying!) This can lead to a fuller discussion of the experience of healing (which is

---

[5] *Ibid.*
[6] Young-Eisendrath and Dawson (1997), glossary, p. 317.
[7] Solomon, Greenberg, and Pyszczynski (1991).

what they are describing) and the role of "depth skills"[8] such as dreamwork or imagework in this process (which they have just experienced).

The Healing Encounter

Findlay's phrase "preparing and holding the space where the miraculous may happen"[9] is a good starting point for this part of the discussion. It reminds us that while the work persona helps to create the right outer and inner environment, the healing, if and when it occurs, is connected to the inner healer and happens as "miracle," in the sense that it cannot be prescribed or willed, or explained in purely rational terms. This is certainly a difficult issue to talk about, not least because the secular vocabulary of healthcare is simply inadequate to describe it.

While acknowledging that there are limits to what we can contribute to the healing process, it is also important to emphasize that there are things we as carers can do to facilitate it. These include an acceptance of our own feelings of helplessness and impotence (which is made easier if we understand the dynamics of countertransference), our being able to wait and trust a process that is happening beyond either party (through the constellation of the wounded healer archetype), and our staying with the person in his or her suffering, without our having to do anything. To return yet again to Findlay's phrase, we "prepare" and we "hold" the space; we do not rush in and fill it with our need to help.

Other issues which arise in discussion on the healing encounter are how it can make the carer more self-aware, how it can change the quality of the subsequent relationship between the carer and the patient, and how it can transform the patient's experience of suffering. Students often speak of how they felt simultaneously healed and aware of their limits or wounds in such an encounter (wounded healers), and describe how their subsequent relationship with the patient became one of friendship, while still being professional. The question of what qualities the patient embodied often reveals an uncanny similarity with those qualities earlier identified in "the healer." This leads to discussion on how the title "wounded healer" applies to *both* the carer *and* the patient in the healing encounter.

---

[8] Kearney (1996), p. 64.
[9] Findlay (1989).

Grounding and Ending

As a way of concluding the workshop, students are asked to spend a few minutes in silence looking at their notes, thinking about the workshop and reflecting on what, if anything, they have learnt. As they do this, they are asked to consider the question:

- "What one small step could I take to incorporate what I have learnt into my work?"

The workshop ends by doing a circle where students share their plan of how they will include their new insight(s) into their clinical practice. This makes it more likely that students will act on what they have experienced.

CHAPTER ELEVEN

An Introductory Workshop on Dreamwork

This is a one-day workshop designed to introduce healthcare professionals to dreamwork. Ideally, this should follow on from the "Whose pain is it anyway?" and "Who am I who cares?" workshops to emphasize that work on self, including ongoing personal work with dreams, is essential groundwork for this approach.

PART 1. SETTING THE CONTEXT

The introductory part of the workshop usually takes the form of a short didactic lecture (using overhead transparencies) outlining the context and theoretical basis for the practice of dreamwork in healthcare. This includes:

- The idea of the containment of care and in particular how this is established by skilled and competent treatment, a relationship of trust between carer and patient and a realization by the carer of the value and necessity of work on self. Emphasis is also placed on dreamwork as an integrated aspect of holistic patient care.

- A brief introduction to Jung's model of the psyche and his ideas on the compensatory function of dreams, the role of archetypes, and the notion of individuation.

- A discussion on attitudes to image, with particular reference to the classical Greek view of dream within the Asklepian as a divine epiphany, an introduction to Hillman's thinking, and a consideration of the implications of Aizenstat's theory of the world unconscious.

- Defining dreamwork in this context as attending to the dream in a way that allows the dream to do its work; a way of working with nature for the healing of suffering.

- Defining the aims of dreamwork as a means of getting to know our patients better, helping patients to better get to know themselves and as a means of offering psychospiritual care. It is emphasized that this form of dreamwork *is not* about dream analysis or dream interpretation.

- Stating the aim of the workshop as being to make students less afraid to listen to their patients' dreams. This is facilitated by students realizing that simply *listening* to another's dreams is itself a valuable and potentially healing form of communication and that this is all that is expected of them.

- Agreeing on possible *indications* for dreamwork through a discussion of the difference between pain and suffering, and curing and healing.

- Discussing *cautions and contra-indications* for dreamwork including issues such as informed consent, confidentiality, and of not working in this way with patients who are acutely confused.

PART 2. LISTENING TO A PATIENT'S DREAM

The students are told that the next part of the workshop will involve listening to a patient's dream and considering how they might respond to this. Initially, they are given the patient's medical and social history with information on the level of awareness he or she has in diagnosis and prognosis, and how he or she appears to be coping at an emotional level. The case history may end like this:

Margaret was readmitted yesterday to the hospital where you are working. It is now early the following morning. You stop by her bedside to say hello and she mentions that she had a "very disturbing dream" last night.

The facilitator then asks the students:

- "How might you as a carer feel on hearing this and how would you respond?"

The students are then asked to join in pairs to discuss this, following which comments are invited from the group. The facilitator begins by focusing on the students' feelings when Margaret mentioned her "very disturbing dream." They often speak of being "taken off guard" and of simply not knowing how to respond. Many describe feelings of anxiety, fear, and panic. Time is taken to discuss such reactions. The facilitator then asks the students how they would respond. The majority of students say they would invite Margaret to talk about her dream, if she would like to. Some qualify this by saying that they would suggest arranging a more suitable time and location to do this. Others speak of how it may be impractical or inappropriate to do this, as for example, when the carer has never met the patient before or knows very little about him or her. Others speak of having neither the desire nor the competence to cope with such a comment from a patient. They describe feelings of inadequacy and their principal concern is how to end this conversation as quickly as possible and in a way that does not unduly upset the patient. All possible responses are discussed and validated, especially the latter. It is essential that students do not feel pressured into participating in something they are not ready or able for. This allows the facilitator to emphasize that dreams are a potent form of information from the unconscious and that it is entirely understandable that healthcare workers with little or no training or experience in this field might feel anxious or inadequate in situations such as this.

If the majority view is to invite Margaret to talk about her dream, the facilitator volunteers to read a previously prepared description. Before actually doing so, he or she invites the students to listen to the dream at "two levels": firstly, to the factual content of the dream and secondly, to notice how they themselves feel on hearing it. The facilitator then reads the dream and, after a short pause, asks:

- "How did you feel on listening to this account and how would you respond?"

The students' feelings are then written on a flip chart. In one such workshop the following feelings were identified at this point: loss, panic, alone, desperation, breathless, fear, terror, heart beating, deep sinking feeling, isolated, separated, sick, out of control, and devastation. As the discussion continued, it became evident that these feelings mirrored how Margaret may well have been feeling at the time of this dream. This allowed for a discussion of how a dream is living unconscious content and how their feeling reaction on hearing it was probably a mixture of their own and Margaret's emotion (ideas on transference and countertransference can also be discussed here).

When looking at how they might then respond, the students need to be reminded that their primary task here is simply to listen and receive the dream, to provide a conscious, holding space for the dream. This is all that is necessary for the patient to remember and truly hear his or her dream and to facilitate the dream's own healing potential. It is common for students to speak of their interesting interpretations and how they feel obliged to share these with the patient. This allows the facilitator to re-emphasize that dreamwork does not mean dream interpretation. Dreamwork means helping a patient to hear his or her dream by listening to it with them. Dreamwork means recognizing that in telling a dream a patient is opening to a process that is already happening and which can bring psychological and spiritual healing. What matters, therefore, is the quality of the carer's listening, rather than anything said or done. The facilitator's refrain should be: "Listen; sit on your interpretations and trust the patient's psyche."

The following schemata may be offered at this point as one possible approach to dreamwork. This can be written on a flip-chart or given to the students as a handout. Time is allowed to discuss each step in detail:

- *Assess:* Is it appropriate to work in this way with this person or not?

- *Explain:* Explain the rationale and logistics of this way of working to the patient.

- *Arrange:* Agree on a time and place.

THE DREAMWORK SESSION ITSELF

Part 1: Opening

- Remind the patient of the rationale and potential benefits of attending to dreams.

- Encourage the patient to describe his or her dream and be aware of your own feelings as you listen.

- Encourage the patient to retell the dream in detail, in the first person, present tense, and be aware of intuitions, images, and daydreams which come as you listen.

- Ask the patient what he or she makes of the dream.

  (It may be appropriate to end the session here. If so, move directly to Part 3. If, on the other hand, it feels appropriate to continue, and if you feel comfortable and competent to do so, move on to Part 2.)

  Part 2: Working With

- Ask the patient about particular dream images that stand out.

- Ask about associations—objective, subjective, and archetypal—to these images.

- Ask the patient to describe certain of these images in detail.

- Be guided in your questioning by interest, curiosity, and intuition.

  Part 3: Closing

- Ask the patient what he or she now makes of the dream.

- Ask, "When you think about your dream and about what's going on in your life at the moment, do you see, or feel, any links, connections, or resonances?"

- Ask, "As you leave the dream and consider what's happening in your life at this time, is there anything you feel you need to do, or say or ask about arising from this?"

- Before ending, encourage the patient to notice and record any feelings or thoughts in the aftermath of the session and to continue to "mull the dream over." The patient may like to continue to work on his or her dream in other creative ways, for example by drawing or painting, either on his or her own or in a session with the art or music therapist. Encourage the patient to record any further dreams. Thank the patient for sharing the dream with you; he or she has literally "bared his or her soul" in the process. Discuss a possible follow-up meeting, if the patient would like this.

PART 3. LISTENING TO EACH OTHERS' DREAMS

The facilitator tells the students that they now have an opportunity to put some of what they have learnt from the previous experience into practice, by listening to one another's dreams. Students are invited to choose a partner and to sit together. They are then instructed to decide which of them will begin as "the dreamer" and which as "the listener." The facilitator has written the following instructions on the flip chart, which he or she explains one at a time:

- The dreamer chooses a dream that feels comfortable to share.

- The listener invites the dreamer to tell his or her dream.

- As the dreamer is telling the dream, the listener notices the factual content *and* how he or she feels on listening to it.

- The listener invites the dreamer to retell the dream in the first person and present tense and with any further details that come to mind.

- This time the listener notices any intuitions, images, or daydreams that come as he or she listens.

- The dreamer then writes down any thoughts or feelings he or she has about the dream while the listener writes down feelings, intuitions, images, or daydreams evoked on listening to it.

- The dreamer shares from the notes he or she has made and on how it was to be listened to in this way. The listener does likewise and shares about how it was to listen in this way.

- The roles are then reversed and the procedure repeated.

PART 4 . PLENARY DISCUSSION

The facilitator now invites the students to reconvene in a plenary group for a general discussion. Open questions are useful at the start, such as:

- "How was it to listen to each others' dreams in this way?"

- "Are there any issues arising from this exercise which anyone would like to discuss?"

The facilitator may also ask the students how they would now feel about listening to a patient's dream. This allows for a review of material covered in the workshop and for the students to raise any outstanding issues they might have. These frequently include the following:

• Students often speak of patients who have a negative or dismissive attitude to any suggestions of dreamwork; such patients may say they have only "rubbishy and unimportant dreams."

Some patients may find it hard to accept the suggestion that dreamwork could be of any value, especially in the context of their being so ill with so many pressing objective needs and concerns. Students may find themselves sharing such feelings, perhaps reflecting a mixture of the counter-transference *and* their own ambivalence about the value of dreamwork.

In discussion it can be pointed out that dreamwork is not some sort of psychological panacea. There are many patients who simply will not want to work in this way and, indeed, it would be entirely inappropriate to in any way cajole or pressurize them to do so against their will. While for some, another approach, such as art therapy, music therapy, or body work may be more acceptable and better suited, others will not want to do anything like this, preferring to stay with more concrete and conventional modes of care.

Another consideration here is that these feelings of ambivalence may be indications of "ego-resistance" on the patient's part to the idea of dreamwork. To paraphrase Francis Bacon, "The ego fears dreamwork as children fear going into the dark." The ego is literally "out of its depth" in dream consciousness where it experiences itself as *not* in control and just one small part of a much bigger story. And so the ego in the waking state and especially in the context of serious illness, resists any attempt to encourage movement towards or into dream consciousness, as in the process of dreamwork. It does this in a psychological version of "flight or fight." Here flight takes the form of moving in the opposite direction to dream consciousness by clinging ever more tightly to rational and literal thinking and to the conviction that only empirical data and objective results are important. Fight, on the other hand, takes the form of undermining the value of dreamwork by implying that this is a trivial pursuit in comparison to the "real" and "serious" tasks on hand. It may be appropriate to discuss Solomon, Greenberg, and Pyszczynski's "terror management theory"[1] at this stage.

The point that patient resistance of this kind must always be respected should be reiterated. It may be the tip of an iceberg of fear, and any attempts to push the patient beyond it could precipitate even greater resistance and increase feelings of insecurity and terror. Such a patient may want and be able to deal with his or her problems only at a literal and objective level, and as that patient's carer one must recognize and acknowledge this. This may, as Saunders puts it, "give that person the security they need to face unsafety"[2] in his or her own time and way. Humility is demanded of the carer at this point and an ability to trust the patient's psyche and his or her choice to deal with the situation in a way that may not be the carer's way. On other occasions the carer will sense a glimmer of openness and must judge whether or not to encourage the patient beyond his or her resistance to at least give dreamwork a try. Such an assessment can be made only in the context of the carer already knowing the patient well and having established a relationship of trust.

A further issue for discussion here is the possibility that the carer's own ambivalence and resistance to dreamwork are being communicated to the patient in the countertransference. Unless one has worked on one's own dreams and has recognized and found ways of living with and through these feelings of ego-resistance in oneself, it is better not to consider working with others in this way. Put positively, the best way of encouraging another from waking consciousness into the depths of dream consciousness is to be familiar with this crossing, and all it entails, oneself. This too will be communicated in the countertransference.

- The issue of drug-induced dreaming is often raised, particularly by doctors and nurses.

This is a real concern as the majority of patients with advanced and incurable illness will be on a host of medications, some of which, such as morphine, are known to affect the rapid eye movement (REM) or dreaming phase of sleep.[3] Certain drugs affect REM sleep by suppressing

---

[1] Solomon, Greenberg and Pyszczynski (1991).
[2] Saunders (1978), p. 6.
[3] Colin M. Shapiro, *ABC of Sleep Disorders* (London, UK: BMJ Publishing Group, 1993), p. 78.

it; others enhance it, which may in turn affect the quality and the content of the dreaming process.[4] There are some occasions where the utterly atypical or psychedelic quality of the dreaming points to a significant pharmacological influence. In such an instance, having listened carefully to the dream, an important aspect of the carer's response will be to explain to the patient what he or she thinks might be happening, combined with a possible adjustment of medication. On other occasions, although there may be a suspicion that the dream-quality is being affected by a drug, it will be clear that the content and feeling tone of the dream is entirely appropriate to what is known of the patient and his or her situation. In other words, the radio is tuned in to the right station even if the volume is a bit higher than usual. Here one would respond to the dream as normal while allowing for the fact that there may be an element of exaggeration or inbuilt amplification owing to the medication.

- Students often ask about "nightmares" with questions like, "What possible value are nightmares?" and, "How can I help someone who is suffering from nightmares?"

Nightmares do seem to be a relatively common occurrence in the setting of serious illness and are often the only reason patients talk about their dreams and that carers come to hear of them.

It is helpful to begin this discussion by asking students to suggest likely causes of nightmares in this context. Students readily identify side-effects of medication or the patient's underlying physical condition as the likeliest causes, and this may well be the case. Such diagnoses may prompt students to suggest the prescription of further medication (night sedation of one kind or another), to suppress the problem and, hopefully, prevent it from recurring. Although it should be emphasized there is always a place for reviewing medication in this situation (which will sometimes mean reducing the dose of a particular drug or changing to an alternative), pharmacological measures should form only a part of a broader response to nightmares and be reserved for those situations where the patient's fear is overwhelming and there is little possibility of responding in a more psychological way. Medication alone as a response to nightmares may prove of very short-term benefit.

---

[4] *Ibid.*, p. 64.

Students may have more difficulty in accepting the idea that nightmares could have a "compensatory" function, that is that they may also come "in the service of wholeness … to help, not harm."[5] Although nightmares are a disturbing and frightening experience for the patient, they may represent a paradoxical rebalancing within the psyche, which ultimately improves that patient's sense of well-being. The difficulty here is the medical model. Operating from this paradigm, carers are so dedicated to the ideal of minimizing distress that it is virtually impossible to imagine something as unpleasant and distressing as a nightmare being in any way helpful for an individual's psychological health. To say more about Jung's theory of the compensatory or homeostatic function of the psyche can be helpful here. This allows students to understand not only why someone who is repressing emotions such as terror, despair, and sadness, perhaps as part of a denial of his or her situation, has a dream that evokes these emotions, but also why he or she *needs* to have such a dream. We must accept that this is a very difficult and unpleasant experience for the patient in the short term, but it may ultimately be of benefit to him or her by facilitating a release of repressed emotion, which might otherwise have done even more damage at a physical or psychological level. Furthermore, by putting him or her more in touch with these emotions, it may produce greater psychological balance and lead to an improved sense of well-being.

It can be of value to then ask the students to think of a simple way of explaining this to the patient. One may say something like,

> Even though this has been a very frightening and unpleasant experience for you, it may, nonetheless, have allowed a release of emotional pressure and actually have been a beneficial, if unpleasant, thing to have happened.

The next step is to encourage the patient to tell his or her dream, perhaps adding that to speak about and share such an experience with another can reduce the distress and fear it has evoked. Sometimes the patient will be too frightened to do this and obviously one accepts their decision while adding, if appropriate, the reassurance that medication can be altered or prescribed to try to ensure that this will not happen again. Occasionally the *dream material* is itself frightening; for example, dreams of being trapped in a hole in the ground and unable to get out.

---

[5] Muff (1996), p. 87.

More commonly it is the *quality of the dream* that is frightening. For example, many patients say that it was the vividness of the dream and the intensity of the feelings it evoked that made them frightened. They may add that it felt "so real" that it left them wondering if it had really happened. Sometimes patients describe finding it difficult to know if they had really wakened because the atmosphere and mood of the dream seemed to linger on into the following day. While patients often find it difficult to talk about their nightmares, they are invariably glad to have done so (they are now no longer isolated in their terror), and usually do not suffer from them again.

PART 5. ENDING

In this final part the facilitator may summarize key aspects of the workshop while reemphasizing certain cautions about working in this way and encouraging students to get further experience in dreamwork. The facilitator may make the following points:

- That a carer should work in this way only if he or she wants to and feels comfortable and competent to do so.

- That dreamwork should occur only within the containment of care and, in particular, within a relationship of trust.

- That the carer should have undergone a basic training in dreamwork and have ongoing experience of working on his or her own dreams. The simplest way of doing this is to begin to keep a dream-journal. One should also seriously consider the possibility of working individually on one's dreams in psychotherapy or with others in a "dream group."

- That the carer should have a sense of the limits of his or her skills and ability in dreamwork and where necessary be prepared to refer on to others more experienced.

- That the carer should be supervised in this area of work by someone experienced in dreamwork and psychotherapy who is familiar with and sympathetic to the concept of dreamwork within healthcare.

SECTION V

PRACTICE

The two case histories recounted in this section are chosen to illustrate an integrated clinical approach, with particular emphasis on Asklepian healing in practice. It is important to emphasize that the following accounts outline only certain aspects of a bigger and more complex story. The context of each of the stories is that of far advanced and terminal illness. The focus in the patients' stories told here is on the Asklepian aspects of their care, but in each instance these were interwoven with ongoing, beneficial Hippocratic treatments. Furthermore, although these stories concentrate on the relationship between each patient and myself as their physician, this was just one of a number of significant relationships these individuals had with different members of the multidisciplinary caring team.

CHAPTER TWELVE

Rosalinda

22 OCTOBER

"I've read *Mortally Wounded* twice, cover to cover, and it brought
me no comfort whatsoever. What am I supposed to do, "wait"? ...
is that *all I* can do?"

Rosalinda had already been in the palliative care unit for almost
two months. We were now meeting to discuss the possibility of
doing some imagework and dreamwork together. I already knew
her well as I had been attending her as a physician and had worked with
the ward team to bring her difficult physical symptoms under control.
About a year previously she had developed severe pain and weakness in
her arms. Extensive investigations had revealed secondary cancer of
unknown origin in the vertebrae of her neck. Orthopedic surgery to
strengthen these bones, followed by a lengthy course of radiotherapy, had
been partially successful in alleviating the pain but the weakness had
persisted unchanged. She was transferred to the palliative care unit in early
July for pain control and rehabilitation in the hope that she would
improve to the point of being able to manage on her own at home again.
She was widowed and had one daughter, Sabha, who was very supportive
to her mother but was not in a position to move back into her mother's
home as carer. Indeed, Rosalinda herself would not have wanted that.

When Rosalinda was admitted to the palliative care unit, she was in great distress. She had constant pain with pins and needles in her arms, hands, and fingers. The power was greatly diminished in both arms and she had lost the ability to perform fine finger movements. In fact, her weakened hands and fingers were already assuming claw-like flexion deformities. Because of her disabilities, she was unable to perform many of the simple tasks of living such as washing, dressing, and attending to her toilet needs. Those of us getting to know her at this stage could not have imagined the woman she had been prior to her illness; by all accounts charming, elegant, and intelligent, renowned for her style and her colourful and successful entertaining. Instead, she was furious, frustrated, and bitter at her predicament. In those early weeks in the unit she focused her rage on different members of the nursing staff in ways that were often cutting and deeply hurtful. At such times it was difficult for many of her carers to make allowances for Rosalinda's behaviour. It often seemed as if she was being horrible simply for the sake of it.

Gradually, over the days and weeks, Rosalinda began to change. She became curious about the people caring for her, particularly the nurses and kitchen staff on the ward. She slowly transformed her single room into "her space," having bits of furniture, pictures, rugs, books, and other treasured objects (including a well-stocked drinks trolley) brought in from home. She began to relax and revealed a dry wit and a wicked sense of humour. Gone were the days when it felt like an ordeal to enter Rosalinda's room on rounds. It was now a pleasure and the danger was of forgetting that we still had another seventeen patients to see besides her; from heart-sinking patient to heart-warming human being. As we sat together in team conference, we took note of this transformation but could not easily explain how and why it had occurred.

Perhaps the change in Rosalinda from the embittered and tortured patient on admission to the enlivening and gracious person she once again became could be seen as a validation of good palliative care. No "one thing," no "one person," no "one intervention" made the difference. It was a combination of multiple small moves and half-moves, relationships of trust built of care and professional skill mixed with a large dose of liking and respect on behalf of the ward team for this fiery, rebellious soul. The way the nurses attended to Rosalinda's needs with patience and gentleness; the constant attention of medical staff to her pain and other physical symptoms; the care with which the kitchen staff organized what and when she wanted to eat and drink; the hours the physiotherapist took to exercise her limp fingers and the sessions he organized for her in the hydrotherapy pool; having her limbs massaged by the aromatherapist and the ongoing work she was doing with the art therapist and the social worker; all these and more were the ingredients which had worked within the alchemical *vas bene clausum* of the unit and its many containing relationships of care to bring about this change.

Rosalinda's asking to meet with me to discuss our doing imagework and dreamwork together was very much her own initiative. This arose from her reading of my working in this way and with encouragement from Deirdre, the art therapist. Deirdre had spoken with me and told me how, as an agnostic, Rosalinda (who was originally from a Roman Catholic background and had been married to a Jew) was feeling very isolated but desperately searching for some spiritual reassurance to counter her terror of death. She added that Rosalinda was also beginning to look at a number of significant issues from her past and present in her art therapy and concluded her comments by saying:

> Rosalinda strikes me as someone who has done a lot of therapy and a lot of talking about herself and her problems in the past. It's like she knows her story really well—yet it seems she's only beginning to get to know herself.

22 October (continued)

I heard Rosalinda's sarcastic humour in her opening comments. I also heard a challenge to me to *do* something tangible to lessen her distress and prove myself as capable in this domain as we had been with her physical pain. I felt it was important to discuss expectations and to look at what might possibly come from our working together in this way. Rosalinda was clear. She wanted certainty; an experience that would confirm that there was an afterlife and that all would be well. She wanted to know this and she wanted to feel this. I said that, much as I would like to, there was no way I could give her this reassurance. I explained that working with the images of our unconscious was a way of "tuning in" to what was going on in our deepest selves; that this was unknown information to our conscious minds which may be of great relevance and significance. It could well be, I added, that she would find what she was searching for by listening carefully to this deep, inner voice, which, in my experience, seemed particularly determined to be heard at times like this. I then asked if she had been dreaming lately. She replied that she could not remember when she had last dreamt, certainly not in recent weeks. Conscious that I may have been falling into a "doing trap" but keen to move beyond this intellectual discussion and enable Rosalinda to experience what this work might entail, I suggested that we do some imagework. She agreed. I asked her to close her eyes and led her through a short introductory centering exercise. I continued:

> "Now, begin to imagine yourself standing on a grassy hill. It's a summer evening and the sun is beginning to set in a clear sky. It's still warm. There is just a very faint breeze, which you feel on your face and in your hair. As you look around, you can see, in the middle distance, a river. It's a large river, wide and obviously deep, because its surface is still and smooth and its black waters hardly appear to be moving. It's coming from hills to one side and you can see it meandering its way to the sea on the far distant western horizon. You look down the hill. You notice that between you and the river is a large green field. You begin to descend through the tall grass towards the river. You know that waiting for you on the bank of the river is someone who knows you and cares deeply about you. You are now getting closer to the river. You can see the person standing there. It may be someone you know well, or it may someone who is unfamiliar to you. You also know that this is someone wise, someone who knows the river and who will be your guide on the next stage of your journey. As you approach this person, he or she greets you. Nearby you notice a little wooden rowing boat tied to the river bank. ... Rosalinda, do you have a sense who this person is?"
>
> "Yes."
>
> "How does it feel to meet this person?"
>
> "I feel I need to ask her forgiveness."
>
> "Imagine yourself doing that. Take your time. Notice how it is to be with the person in this way and what happens. ... And if this person were to invite you to step into the boat with her, how would that be?"
>
> "I think I trust her ... I feel I should ... but I don't want to get in."

Rosalinda was looking troubled as she said this and she had begun to cry. I said:

> "Maybe this is about meeting this person rather than getting into the boat. It's all right to leave it here. If it's OK with you, begin to say goodbye to this person for now and when you are ready open

your eyes and come back to this room and this time where we can talk about what's happened."

"It was Kate, from Mayo. She used to live with her brother but then she came to live with us in Sligo to help Mamma. That was before I was born. I was closer to her than I was to my mother. She wasn't attractive. She had stubble on her chin and her hair in plaits, like one of those Sacred Heart pictures. She wasn't physically affectionate but I was very close to her and she to me. She had a great sense of herself. And she was very close to nature. She had a way with animals and they loved her. "Mousy," she would say in the kitchen. The mouse would come out from behind the cupboard and she'd hit it dead with a broom! And she had this running battle with this big yellow rat that used to sit on the garden wall. They used to look at each other. I can never have new potatoes without thinking of her. When I returned from living in America she was living with Mamma in Dublin. I wanted to see a lot of her but she died soon after. When I was in the States, she used to send me *Ireland's Own* magazine every week. I loved her but I was a bit ashamed of her and I feel bad about that. I can't imagine her by a river ... the sea maybe but more so in a field and with plants. She had this amazing connection with nature."

"If Kate was with you now, Rosalinda, what would this give you?"

She did not answer but began to weep. Then she began to tell more stories about Kate and said she had been thinking about her a lot recently. I spoke of the value of remembering and said that the fact that she felt Kate so close to her at this time seemed significant. I was especially struck by her description of Kate's "great sense of herself" and of her closeness to nature through the land and plants and animals. I shared these thoughts with Rosalinda and quoted Marie-Louise von Franz's words, that, if we allow it to, "Nature through dreams, prepares us for death."[1] I suggested to her that she might begin to record any dreams she had in a journal or on a dictaphone and that, if she would like, we could meet again like this at the same time next week. She said she would like this.

That night I had the following dream:

There is this older woman with a piece of furniture outside her house. I am there also. It's an old, antique, Victorian couch. The woman is discovering that inside the couch are some ants and I'm thinking, "Not surprising really considering it has been in India."

---

[1] von Franz (1987), p. vii.

> There's a little tear in the seat part and she's trying to flick the insects out with a finger but then I'm shocked at her deliberateness as she puts a hand in and deliberately pulls a wedge back opening it right up. (As she's doing this I'm wondering how she'll manage to put it together again.) I look over her shoulder, expecting to see lots of ants in there. In fact, it's full of maggots and worms—lively, healthy, intertwined, and slimy. She then pulls open yet another part to the right side of the couch and it's also teeming with worms. She starts to scoop them out. By now, I'm standing behind the couch with a piece of paper kitchen towel in my hands. I'm wondering how much to intervene to help her. I'm not really doing a lot. What she's doing is enough. Besides I don't really want to.

I knew on waking that this was a dream about Rosalinda. I wondered about the significance of her appearance in this way. She was not dreaming (or at least not remembering her dreams), yet here I was dreaming about her. The dream imagery seemed to be an accurate description of the work she was undertaking and of my sense of inadequacy in her presence. Was this an aspect of countertransference, such that I was dreaming for her? And should I share this with her and see how she responded? I felt instinctively that the answer to this was "no" and that I should keep this to myself.

28 OCTOBER

On rounds Rosalinda was in good form. As a result of decisions made in art therapy she had arranged for a valuable rug to be placed into storage and had a smaller rug and some other artifacts of great sentimental value brought in from home to decorate her room. She was pain free and said that, in contrast to the previous weeks, she had begun to sleep the nights through.

29 OCTOBER

As I approached Rosalinda's room for our scheduled meeting I was aware that I was feeling anxious. I asked myself; "If Rosalinda hasn't dreamt, what will we do?" I had heard from Deirdre that the art therapy session that morning "hadn't gone far"; if anything she felt that Rosalinda had moved backwards from where she had been some weeks previously.

Initially, Rosalinda spoke again of Kate and how she was interested that it was she who had appeared to her in the imagework. As she spoke I noticed that I was feeling bored and a bit lost. I asked her if she had

had any dreams and she said no, qualifying this by saying, "I sensed that Mamma was nearby, on the edge of my dreams." I suggested that if she would like it we could do more imagework. She agreed. As I led her through an initial relaxation procedure, her phone rang. It was Sabha; she would ring her back. Rosalinda left her phone off the hook and I invited her to close her eyes and to imagine the following scene:

> "You are walking through a field. You can feel the grass against your legs. It is a warm summer's evening. Ahead of you is a forest. You are approaching the forest and as you come closer you can see an opening in the trees. There is a pathway there leading into the forest. You pause and consider: *Do I want to enter the forest?* Notice how you are feeling."

> "No, I don't want to enter the forest. I'm frightened."

> "That's OK. Nearby where you are standing, you see a small rock in the sun. You could sit on this if you chose. As you wait there, you know that shortly a wise creature of the forest, some gentle, ancient being, is going to emerge and approach you. You hear a rustle. The creature is emerging and approaching you. Notice the creature as it comes close, how it greets you. Be aware of how you feel. Ask yourself if there is anything you want to say or do. Notice what is happening. … Then, when you are ready, begin to prepare to leave. Find a way to say goodbye and come back to the here and now."

As Rosalinda opened her eyes, I asked her to describe what had happened during the imagework:

> "The very sight of the forest freaked me. I felt frightened and panicky. There was no way I could go in there. And I hate myself for this. I know I *should* be able to "go with the flow" and I want to, but I can't. I always have to control everything. The only time I ever could was a number of years ago when I was on Prozac for eighteen months. … Then I left the path around a clump of trees. The first rock was too big but I found one nearby that I could sit on. From there I could see down the valley. It reminded me of a wonderful picnic we went on many years ago. Sabha was with me. It was near Mountrath in County Laois. It rained but we were very happy. I wish heaven could be like that . . ."

> "And did a creature emerge from the forest?"

> "Yes. At first I thought it was a donkey but its hooves were soft rather than hard, more like a cat or a bear. It was a wild creature, gentle, like Sabha's deer. I just wanted to hold it, to feel its softness, to feel it nuzzle into me."

Her mention of deer reminded me of some I had seen the previous weekend in a forest near Killarney. I told Rosalinda of this encounter and asked her why she referred to "Sabha's deer." She then told me the myth of Sadbh, the beautiful deer-princess of ancient Ireland and beloved of Finn McCool. This was the first time I had heard this story and yet part of it bore an uncanny resemblance to a powerful dream I had some years previously. I felt a shiver of recognition as I listened.

Following this session I began to consider suggesting to Rosalinda that she consult the *I Ching*, the ancient Chinese oracle, and that we might take time to look at this together at our next meeting. I had recently been reading about this 3000-year-old method of accessing the archetypal aspects of the unconscious and had become very interested in it.

In my reading I had learned how the *I Ching* had been popularized in the West by Jung through his familiarity with the translation of his friend, missionary and sinologist Richard Wilhelm. In 1949, in the foreword Jung wrote for Wilhelm's translation of the *I Ching*, he identified the assumption that underpins the oracle:

> This assumption involves a certain curious principle that I have termed synchronicity, a concept that formulates a point of view diametrically opposed to that of causality. Since the latter is a merely statistical truth and not absolute, it is a sort of working hypothesis of how events evolve one out of another, whereas synchronicity takes the coincidence of events in space and time as meaning something more than mere chance, namely, a peculiar interdependence of objective events among themselves as well as with the subjective (psychic) states of the observer or observers.
>
> The ancient Chinese mind contemplates the cosmos in a way comparable to that of the modern physicist, who cannot deny that his model of the world is a decidedly psychophysical structure. The microphysical event includes the observer just as much as the reality underlying the *I Ching* comprises subjective, i.e., psychic conditions in the totality of the momentary situation. Just as causality describes the sequence of events, so synchronicity to the Chinese mind deals with the coincidence of events.[2]

I had also encountered Rudolf Ritsema and Stephen Karcher's translation of the *I Ching*[3] and been impressed by their description of

---

[2] Carl G. Jung, Foreword, in Richard Wilhelm, *I Ching or Book of Changes* (London, UK: Arkana, 1989), p. xxiv.

[3] Rudolf Ritsema and Stephen Karcher, *I Ching* (Dorset, UK: Element, 1994).

how the oracle could be used as a tool to put one in touch with the deeper workings of the psyche:

> The *I Ching* ... is a particular kind of imaginative space set off for a dialogue with the gods or spirits, the creative basis of experience now called the unconscious. An oracle translates a problem or question brought to it into an image language like that of dreams. It changes the way you experience the situation to connect you with the inner forces that are shaping it. The oracle's images dissolve what is blocking the connection, making the spirits available. ... It puts you back into what the ancients called the sea of the soul by giving advice on attitudes and actions that lead to the experience of imaginative meaning.[4]

> Antique civilization, both East and West, used divination and oracle to keep in contact with unseen powers. ... The idea that words, things and events can become omens that open communication with a spirit-world is based on an insight into the way the psyche works—that in every symptom, conflict or problem we experience there is a spirit trying to communicate with us. Each encounter with trouble is an opening to this spirit, usually opposed by the ego because it wants to enforce its will on the world. Divination gives a voice to what the ego has rejected. It brings up the hidden complement or shadow of the situation in order to link you with the myths and spirits behind it. This changes the way you see yourself, your situation and the world around you.[5]

> The *I Ching* is meant to be used when you are troubled and you seek a meaning in the disturbance ...
> Using the *I Ching* in this way is like working with dreams. The images do not offer standard predictions of an unalterable future. They describe the way energy is moving to create possible futures. This presents you with an opportunity to interact with the energy clusters or complexes of the psyche. Changing your relation to these forces can change what will happen to you.
> Perhaps the most fundamental quality of the Oracle is to recognize and act as a witness to your situation. This grounds you in an image that is larger than your personal awareness. Such recognition is the basic connection to the symbolic world.[6]

It seemed, therefore, that consulting the *I Ching* was an ancient Chinese method of helping an individual to "go with the flow." In the terminology of the *I Ching,* it did this by helping that person to recognize

[4] *Ibid.*, p. 8.
[5] *Ibid.*, pp. 10-11.
[6] *Ibid.*, pp. 32-33.

and get "in Tao," which literally meant "the way," that is "the flow or stream of creative energy that makes life possible, the way *in which* everything happens and the *way on which* everything happens."[7] Related to the word *Tao* was the word *te,* "often translated as power or virtue, [and] refer[ing] to the power to realise *Tao* in action to become what you are meant to be"; while a *chün tzu* was someone who sought to acquire *te* through divination, to live connected to the *Tao;* "What the *chün tzu* finds through this dialogue is significance, the experience of spirit, meaning and connection."[8]

All of this seemed pertinent to Rosalinda's situation. Given the absence of spontaneous dreaming, perhaps this ancient method of "experimental dreaming" had something to offer.

30 OCTOBER

Meanwhile, there was a general feeling on the ward that Rosalinda had become calmer and was less demanding. She had mentioned to one of the nurses that she was feeling "more hopeful than she had been." When we called in to see her on rounds, she spoke of how it was her husband's anniversary. He had died of a cerebrovascular accident in New York when Sabha was just a few weeks old. She also spoke of how her mother had also died in the hospice and wondered at the irony of them both, so unalike in all kinds of ways, having this experience in common.

As the others left the room I stayed behind to introduce the idea to Rosalinda of consulting the *I Ching* at our next session. I asked her if she was familiar with this way of working. She replied that all she knew was that it was some form of fortune-telling, "like studying tea-leaves or flocks of birds." I agreed that although this was its popular image, a more accurate description was as a way to discern "how the currents were moving in the river of the unconscious" and that in this it was closer to dreaming than gazing into a crystal ball. I gave her some literature, which I had photocopied, on the history, theory, and methodology of the *I Ching* and suggested that she have a look at this before we next met. She could then decide if she was interested in this proposal.

---

[7] *Ibid.,* p. 10.
[8] *Ibid.*

5 November

Rosalinda had had a fall in the bathroom the previous night. She had lost her balance when bending forward at the sink, pulled upright but then fallen back on her bottom. Apparently she had been very shaken by this accident and had taken a long time to settle. On waking she was still sore. When I arrived for our session she was in bed and looked sleepy. She had recently had some quick-acting morphine tablets for her pain. She was reading the papers I had given her on the *I Ching*. She said she was finding it hard to understand, so once again I attempted to explain how I saw it and how I felt it might help her:

> I see the *I Ching* working like our dreams in that both can help us tune in to what is happening in the deep, unconscious parts of our psyches. It's not so much about black and white answers as a collection of images in which we can recognize and reflect on our own situation. This may bring us a degree of insight and a sense of connectedness to what is happening.

Rosalinda was looking at me heavy-lidded, nodding occasionally. I was very aware of her tiredness and of how excited I was to try this way of working. I knew I had to be careful not to impose something on her she neither understood nor wanted. I asked her what she thought. She replied that she was keen to go ahead.

I then explained that the first and very important step was for her to decide how she was going to frame her question. I asked her what question she would like to ask, suggesting that she imagine she now had the opportunity to ask a wise and compassionate being anything she wished. She thought about this for a while and replied that she would like information on life after death. When I asked her to put this as a question, she replied:

> "What do I need to do to get ready for death?"

Next I explained that the method we were going to use in performing the *I Ching* involved her choosing coloured marbles from a bag and explained the four different types of lines that could result and go to form the hexagram.

> "If anyone looks in they'll conclude that we're definitely losing our marbles!" Rosalinda quipped as she reached into the bag.

The primary hexagram was 54, called *Converting the Maiden;* with a moving yang line in the second place, this changed to the related hexagram 51, called *Shake/Arousing.* I explained that while the primary hexagram was said to describe the present situation and the transforming lines particular "hot spots" in this, the related hexagram was said to comment on how the present situation would develop in time. I suggested I read out each of these three texts and we could then take time to discuss them. I also said I would photocopy the texts and leave them with her to read over at her leisure if she so wished:

> 54, Converting the Maiden:
> *Keywords: Realize hidden potential. Let yourself be led.*
> Converting the maiden describes your situation in terms of a change you must go through which is beyond your control. You are not the one who has chosen. The force involved is larger than you are. The way to deal with it is to accept it and let yourself be led. You cannot escape your situation. It reflects a deep and unacknowledged need. It is moving you towards a new field of activity, the place where you belong. Don't try to discipline people or take control of the situation. That will cut you off from the spirits and leave you open to danger. Don't impose your will, have a plan and a place to go. Being free of such plans will bring you profit and insight. This is a very special situation that, in the long run, can lead to great success.[9]

As I read this slowly, Rosalinda was listening intently and nodding occasionally. When I finished, she asked me to read through it again, which I did. Then she commented:

> "It seems to be telling me to 'let go,' but how do I do that?"

> "I see this as happening already, Rosalinda, more and more. It's what I see today; you are allowing the bed to hold your bruised body. In this you and your body are trusting what's happening."

> "Like hoping. I'm hopeful ... is it safe to hope?"

> "I'm not sure about safe, in fact it's probably a lot safer not to hope; perhaps the safest place of all would be a black hole of hopelessness. But it's human and it's courageous ... hope opens you ... in that sense it makes you more vulnerable."

I then read the transforming line:

---

[9] Stephen Karcher, *The I Ching* (Dorset, UK: Element, 1995), pp. 157-158.

Nine at the second: By squinting at things you will be able to see them. Take an independent perspective. Looking at things from solitude and obscurity brings profit and insight. The rules aren't changing yet. *Direction:* There is a fertile shock on the way. Re-imagine the situation. Gather energy for a decisive new move.[10]

Rosalinda asked me to read the second or related hexagram as well at this stage. I continued:

51, Shake/Arousing:
Keywords: The shock of the new. Stir things up. Don't get flustered.
Shake/Arousing describes your situation in terms of a disturbing and inspiring shock. The way to deal with it is to rouse things to new activity. Re-imagine what you are confronting. Let the shock shake up your old beliefs and begin something new. Don't get flustered. Don't lose your depth and concentration. What at first seems frightening will soon be a cause to rejoice. This is pleasing to the spirits. Through it they will give you success, effective power and the capacity to bring the situation to maturity. The thunder rolls and everyone is frightened. You can hear them screaming in terror. Then the fright changes to joy and you hear everyone laughing and talking. The sudden shock spreads fear for thirty miles around. Don't lose your concentration. Hold the libation cup calmly so the dark wine arouses and calls the spirits.[11]

"Well," began Rosalinda, "I suppose death is a bit of a 'shaking up.' a 'shock.'"

We talked on for some time about these readings and she asked to me reread certain parts. We noted that while this second hexagram spoke of fear it also seemed to be pointing to joy and even laughter beyond this. I reflected that:

"Letting go doesn't mean 'no fear.' On the contrary, there may be fear and perhaps sadness and confusion. But the hexagram speaks of something beyond the fear also ... "

I was amazed by how relevant the various texts of the reading seemed to be to Rosalinda's situation. Despite being so broad-ranging, I was also struck by how she was able to focus on those aspects of the readings that interested her and which she was ready for and wanted to look at. It had allowed us to consider something different together and to talk about

---

[10] *Ibid.*, p. 159.
[11] *Ibid.*, pp. 150-151.

familiar issues with an honesty and directness that felt valuable. Shortly
afterwards, when I returned with the photocopied pages, I found
Rosalinda deeply asleep.

12 NOVEMBER

I met with Deirdre, the art therapist, over lunch to discuss our mutual
work with Rosalinda. She had had a session that morning when Rosalinda
had finished a collage she had been working on. This included a pair of
miniature shoes, which Rosalinda had painted gold and which were facing
diagonally upwards towards the top left-hand corner of the piece. These
shoes were surrounded with tiny green plastic toy soldiers, guns pointed
as if under attack. The background colours were blues of different shades.
There were various natural artifacts, seeds, tiny leaves, glued on in different
places and across the top of the piece was a swirling cloud of lace and glitter
of many different colours. Deirdre felt that Rosalinda was working well
and that this piece, as with other things she had done, showed a wonderful
sense of colour and design. She also wondered at the fact that the direction
of the golden shoes was upwards where most of the content and activity
of the piece was also located. Was there something here about getting above
and beyond the earthly and the mundane? Deirdre also mentioned that
Rosalinda had told her of a dream she had had the previous afternoon,
which she was keen to tell me. Without recounting the dream, she said it
fitted with her sense that Rosalinda was yet again on a threshold and
engaging with the implications of this.

Rosalinda was sitting in the armchair next to her bed. She was drowsy
but in no pain. The drowsiness was annoying her. It was probably due
to the increase in her analgesia following her recent fall, which could now
be reduced. I reassured her of this. She also spoke of her worries about
the increasing stiffness and diminishing use of her hands. Since she had
had a further course of radiotherapy to her neck following her admission
to the palliative care unit, was already wearing a neck support collar,
having maximum physiotherapy, and on corticosteroids, there were few
if any outstanding treatment possibilities. The only pharmacological
option was to further increase the steroids. Rosalinda knew that this move
was possible but she was not keen, mainly because of the potential
cosmetic side-effects of the steroids. She knew, nonetheless, that this
intervention was available should things get really bad. Then she began
to tell me about the previous afternoon:

"A friend took me out to Powerscourt. It was a beautiful autumn day. The sky was blue and clear. The air was cold. The remaining leaves on the trees were golden. The gardens were wonderful and we spent some time in the shop and had a cup of tea. I was exhausted on my return and slept. I had the following dream:

I am on the landing in the old Powerscourt house, on the first floor. I'm in a wheelchair. It's so beautiful, so spacious and full of light. The walls are a soft orange colour and sprinkled with gold dust with azure blue coming through in places. Doorways are inlaid into the walls. There's a sense of luminosity, of warmth, of beauty. At either side of the landing there are these curved stairwells that lead to the ground floor. They're made of scrubbed white stone. Each step is shallow and spaced. I go down the right stairwell and I'm expecting a bumpy ride but in fact it's amazingly smooth and easy. I look back on reaching the ground and realize that it is smooth, like a ramp, even though it had looked like steps from above. I'm in the hallway so I can look out the front door. Outside it's misty and it begins to rain. There's a young man there. He's tall, thin, a bit uptight, some gray hair. He steps into the portico opposite, sort of half out of the rain. I call to him to come in out of the rain but he turns and looks at me with a bit of scowl of disapproval as if he's shrugging off the suggestion … I'm not sure, but he may have been helping me earlier with my wheelchair."

"Any thoughts or feelings about Powerscourt?" I asked.

"Not really," Rosalinda replied and continued, "While the gardens there are beautiful—and come to think of it yesterday's colours were there in the dream in the walls of the first floor landing—it's *too* perfect. Humans look very small in it. It's not the sort of place children might play in. If that's what heaven's going to look like, I don't like it very much. Too cold, clinical, inhuman."

"Was there any sense that you were about to leave the house?"

"No, the sense is that I want the young man to come in from the rain for his sake. … I'm being fussy."

"What if it's about being in the house, staying there?"

"I'd like that. It's so beautiful, warm, luminous, spacious."

"And what about the young man?"

"He's about your height. He reminds me a bit of someone I know, the same figure as him. I used to think he disapproved of me and my parties when I first knew him. He is very religious … in the good sense; thoughtful, looks out for others. In recent years I have come to like him … "

"Is that sense of disapproval familiar to you?"

"Oh yes, I often feel like that. Yesterday, Sabha told me that her partner, Noel, loved me. I was surprised and delighted. I wasn't so sure about him at first ... I don't like thick hair in a man. He's quiet, reserved. But I like him more and more as I've got to know him. He's so kind."

"While dreams can use material from our outer world, and this is apparent in the way your dream incorporated elements of your actual visit to Powerscourt yesterday, they can also be a snapshot of our inner world at that moment. If that is true, can you feel any resonances between the dream and what's happening for you these times?"

"Maybe I'm coming to know this inner experience I've been looking for."

"Yes, I was wondering about that also. I believe our dreams aren't just about understanding in the sense of something we "hunt down" and "get." They are also about the actual experience of the dream itself. For me, there's also something here about appreciating that while dreams happen "in me" they're not entirely "of me." In some essential way dreams are already complete in themselves, they don't need either my approval or my reason in this. I'm reminded of how you described Kate."

"Funny you remember Kate. I've been thinking a lot of her. Her mole, her bristles, ... but such a complete person in herself. I don't know what she'd make of Powerscourt. I do know she wouldn't have been in the least phased by it. ... I was also thinking of a golden globe, like a Christmas decoration, not circular, more spheroidal ... a bit of an onion shape, with layers of gold and blue. I remember seeing this exhibition in Boston; the artist painted only onions, she was able to capture that luster on a peeled onion's skin. ... I wish I had dreamt of Kate."

"Maybe Kate is part of those dream images. It certainly sounds as though she had some of that golden wholeness."

"Yes."

As I prepared to leave I thanked Rosalinda for sharing the story of Sadbh with me and told her that I had later read the full version of the myth,[12] and found it was wonderful. I asked her if she had any further

---

[12] Marie Heaney, *Over Nine Waves: A Book of Irish Legends* (London, UK: Faber & Faber, 1994), pp. 171-179.

thoughts on the I *Ching* reading. She said she had been too tired to do any reading in the meantime. I had already explained that I would be away the following week and it was planned that she could have an additional art therapy session if she so wished. I asked if there was anything I could do before I left. She asked me to turn on her lamp with its orange lampshade behind her. A soft, warm golden light surrounded Rosalinda. I sensed she could allow herself to be held in this.

26 NOVEMBER

Before my meeting with Rosalinda I had been lecturing a group of nurses on "the management of the confused patient." While delivering the lecture, something had caught my eye. To my right, on a cupboard at the top of the lecture theatre, was a pair of life-size golden shoes resting on a red satin cushion. I was stunned by this and immediately thought of Rosalinda's collage. An hour later, as I went through the door of her room, I saw this displayed on the wall. It was more colorful and beautiful than I had imagined. As we began, I told Rosalinda of the "coincidence" with the golden shoes and admired her collage. She said that her work with Deirdre was going really well and she had met with her twice weekly while I was away. She spoke of how happy she was these times and less and less wanting to die:

> "I had one year when I was as happy as this before in my life, the first year of my marriage ... and I'm feeling less of a burden on Sabha."

I asked if she had any dreams in the interim and she said she had not. It was evident that she wanted to talk and she ranged from topic to anecdote to memory to questions:

> "I've been wondering again about life after death. I've one friend who believes that the spirit of the dead person stays around afterwards until it finds an empty womb. I don't like the sound of that. When the Little Mermaid dies at the end of that story, she changes form and joins the heavenly chorus around the world. ... I hope it's like that. What do you think?"

> "I've no idea how it will be but I do believe that life continues in some way. People I've worked with who have been approaching death often describe a growing sense of life and hope even as their body is fading. I don't think these feelings and the sorts of images and experience that come through dreams and art at a time like this

are just some cruel joke life is playing on us. I believe, as
Wordsworth put it, they are 'Intimations of Immortality.'"

I asked Rosalinda if she ever had such a pair of golden shoes herself.
She began talking of the early days of her marriage to Nathan and how
he had treated her so well with all kinds of beautiful clothes and jewelry.
Then she spoke of financial difficulties that had arisen after his death
because of an unmade will. She returned to speaking about Nathan
himself and her enormous pain and frustration that Sabha never had the
opportunity to get to know her father. She mused on how wonderful it
would be if he were around to help Sabha at this time and added:

> "Well, maybe he is with her. She certainly has many of his qualities.
> … I just wish I could let him go … "

3 DECEMBER

I met with Deirdre before seeing Rosalinda. She told me of a mobile
Rosalinda had just completed. Her sense was that although there was
something celebratory in what Rosalinda was doing in her art, she was
also worried about the danger of her losing contact with reality. I
wondered if this creative activity might also be a concretizing of her
unconscious process. Perhaps Rosalinda was, to quote D. H. Lawrence,
"building her ship of death,"[13] collating and assembling materials for a
soul vessel, which could survive her body's demise and carry her spirit
onwards?

As I said hello to Rosalinda she handed me a brochure for an
exhibition by the artist Clodagh Redden that had recently opened and
which she hoped to visit with Deirdre. In the programme I read that the
exhibition featured boats "in which the souls travel through the nether
regions between life and death," an exhibition of "ships of death"! I told
her of the coincidence of this with my thoughts about her own work.
Suspended from the ceiling of her room was a branch with many spindled
arms from which brightly coloured houses, trees, balloons, and angels
hung. I admired this and asked her how she was feeling:

> "More and more frightened … and my hands are getting worse.
> I'm frightened of death as an 'abyss.' I came across this article in
> Saturday's *Irish* Times where I read this: 'Comatose and connected

---

[13] Lawrence (1993), p. 961.

by a dozen tubes to a dozen machines, Mark hovered in a "pre-
morbid state," the medical term for the edge of the abyss.' That
makes me think of going down into nothingness. ... I'd rather go
up to heaven."

I asked Rosalinda if she had any dreams. She replied:

"Yes, last night and not very pleasant:

I am walking in this gray mud. It's twilight. It's like in the trenches
in the First World War. I'm alone ... but I know it's to do with this
man I had an affair with for many years. I feel deeply ashamed,
trapped, frightened."

Rosalinda's face was screwed up as she spoke. It was evident that it
was painful and difficult for her to talk about it. I asked her if she would
like to say more about this. She spoke about an affair she had when she
was fourteen with a much-trusted family friend, a married middle-aged
man. She described how she wanted to get out of this and realized that
if she became pregnant she would be "trapped." She knew her mother
suspected what was going on but she could never prove it. The affair
ended only when Rosalinda fell in love with another, even older, man.
She was in tears as she spoke and concluded by saying:

"I'm so deeply ashamed of this. I'd thought I'd dealt with it ... "

"And if some of these feelings related to your present situation, can
you feel any connections?"

"Oh yes! I feel very ashamed of so much ... "

Again and again Rosalinda moved off into other anecdotes and
memories, many amusing, all interesting. However, my feeling was that
it was important to stay with the dream and so I asked:

"Mud, trapped, fear?"

"I felt so trapped in the affair."

"Any mud around these days?"

"Oh yes ... these hands."

I spoke of Jung's theory that although dreams like this are painful
and difficult, they may also be beneficial in some not very obvious ways;
that they could help to bring in feelings and memories which are necessary
to restore balance and wholeness to our psyches. Rosalinda responded:

"Like pieces of a jigsaw? If I could see it like that, I'd feel better. I
see it as stuff I'd dealt with coming back to haunt me. Stuff I need
to let go of but can't."

Once again, Rosalinda was in tears. I said:

"Rosalinda, you've given it space today; maybe that was what was
necessary."

"Let's just hope there's no more mud … "

As I prepared to leave, Rosalinda asked if I knew the Flanders and
Swann song about mud and started to sing:

Mud, mud, glorious mud,
Nothing quite like it for cooling the blood,
So follow me, follow me down to the hollow
For there we can wallow in glorious mud!

I left her room smiling and with feelings of deep affection for this
colorful and courageous soul.

10 December

Since I had last seen her, Rosalinda had been interviewed for a
television documentary that was being made about the work of the
hospice. She impressed the producer of the programme as "a woman who
was utterly herself." By then her room was looking amazing. This was a
result of her combined efforts with a designer friend and the work she
had done with Deirdre in her most recent sessions. Huge serpentine
swathes of green and red material coiled around the curtains as her mobile
caught the light of the many candles burning around the room. She
herself looked radiant:

"I think at times recently I'm happier than I've ever been in my
life … am I euphoric on the morphine?"

"No you're not. When you're on the dose of morphine you need
for your pain, you may be very happy to be out of pain but you're
not 'euphoric.'"

"I'm glad to hear this. … I've been thinking a lot of Mamma
recently, but not dreaming of her, I wish I could … "

Rosalinda then reminisced at length about her mother, who had been a
midwife and the matron of a hospital in Sligo. She and Rosalinda had fought
constantly and there had obviously been a lot of rivalry between them.

"She could never allow for the fact that I was prettier than her. She used to say I was 'passable.' After my husband died, Mamma wrote to me and said, 'You've had it all, marriage, money, a child—now come home to me.' Instead, my sister went to live with her. ... When she came into the hospice in 1984 she was ninety. At first she was as crotchety as ever but when she was given enough morphine to take away her pain she became a changed person. She was nice again, like she was when we were very young. But she was ambitious and as her career took off she changed. ... She used to tell me that I was her favourite."

"Why would you like to dream of your mother? What would you like to hear from her? What do you imagine that might give you?"

"To know that I'm her favourite ... to know that she really meant it. This raft I'm on, though the waters rise from time to time ... to know that would make me feel more secure. Yet Kate was the one who came. Kate was there as my guide on the way across. ... I could have two, couldn't I?"

Rosalinda then spoke again about Kate and about the tangible yet undemonstrative bond between them. Kate had died in the 1970s, within a year of Rosalinda's returning to Ireland from North America.

"She died in St James's hospital; I crashed the car on my way to see her that day. She had such a wonderful affinity with animals. Saint Francis with bad thoughts! 'Mousy,' ... Wallop! And that big yellow rat on the garden wall with his scarred face and a lame paw from a trap ... he and Kate were sworn enemies, and admirers. ... If only I could dream of Mamma ... "

"When did you last see your mother?"

"On the day she died, which was the sixth of February 1984. I looked into the room where she had been moved. I remember the bare white walls. There were two aunts sitting with her. I didn't feel I had a place, so I didn't go in. Instead I visited a friend who was in the Rehabilitation Hospital in Dun Laoghaire. They phoned me there to tell me she'd died."

"Would you like to do some imagework around that final visit?"

"No." [screwing up her face] "No, I'd like to. Pass me the tissues."

"Close your eyes and take some time to rest in yourself ... now begin to remember, if you can, how it was as you approached your mother's room that day. You look in the door. Your mother is lying there. There is no one else there. She hasn't seen you yet. Notice how she looks. Notice how you feel. When you're ready, find a way to greet her. Pull over a chair and sit by her. Say and do whatever you want and need to do. ... Notice how she responds."

At this stage Rosalinda was in great distress, weeping and moaning.

> "Rosalinda, stay with how you are feeling ... notice how your
> mother responds to you ... when you are ready and if this feels
> complete, find a way to take your leave for now and begin to come
> back to the here and now ... You obviously loved your mother very
> much."

> "So much ... and she was so beautiful ... the nun on the ward said
> she was like the Virgin Mary."

> "Would you like to describe what happened for you there?"

> "I knelt at her bedside ... I laid my head on her breast ... I said I
> was sorry for so many things. ... She put her arms around me."

> "Did she say anything?"

> "Something like, 'It's all right ... ' If only I could have done this at
> the time. ... If only those two women weren't there. ... The room
> was so white and bare. Such a contrast to this one! And I fought
> with her the whole time. ... She was unreliable; surely that's the
> worst thing you can say about your mother. And yet she was so
> reliable as a midwife. The people in Sligo used to talk of her as a
> 'white witch.' They used to say she had magic. A very complex
> woman ... she just shouldn't have had her own children; she'd have
> been a great aunt! ... Thank you."

It felt to me that this session had been very difficult for Rosalinda.
My task had been to try to allow her to be, in her suffering (without
rushing in with the tissues—or the kitchen towel for that matter!—real
or metaphorical) and in her grief for her mother. Earlier I had been
reminded of a piece I had read by novelist Harold Brodkey, which he
wrote shortly before his death from AIDS. I told Rosalinda about this
and dropped a copy of it into her the following day. The final paragraph
read:

> One may be tired of the world—tired of the prayer-makers, the
> poem-makers, whose rituals are distracting and human and pleasant
> but worse than irritating because they have no reality—while reality
> itself remains very dear. One wants glimpses of the real. God is an
> immensity, while this disease, this death, which is in me, this small,
> tightly defined pedestrian event, is merely and perfectly real,
> without miracle—or instruction. I am standing on an unmoored
> raft, a punt moving on the flexing, flowing face of a river. It is
> precarious. I don't know what I am doing. The unknowing, the taut

balance, the jolts and the instability spread in widening ripples through all my thoughts. Peace? There was never any in the world. But in the pliable water, under the sky, unmoored, I am traveling now and hearing myself laugh, at first with nerves and then with genuine amazement. It is all around me.[14]

17 DECEMBER

This was to be our last meeting before Christmas.

"I want to tell you this dream I had last night," Rosalinda announced. "I walked into my bathroom where I had stored all my Christmas gifts for everyone in the empty bath. It was full of bottles of wine, boxes of chocolate and lots of other things. But someone had run the water and everything was wet. It looked as if a lot of the stuff was ruined but maybe some of it was salvageable. I knew it was Nora [one of the nurses caring for her] who had done this. I was dismayed but it was also like I'd been expecting it."

I asked Rosalinda what her thoughts and feelings around the dream were. She replied:

"As soon as I got to the door of the bathroom I knew it had happened even before I saw it. The bottoms of the gifts were in the water. They squelched. And I knew it was Nora. And then this sense of dismay, disappointment, and inevitability. I love Nora. We get on really well. She reminds me of so many women from the West of Ireland—strong, direct, warm, life-giving. ... No, this is just like what Mamma would do. She'd let me go so far and then tell me I'd gone too far, that I was being 'actressy,' as she used to say, and pull the ground out from under my feet. Bursting the bubble. I've been almost too good recently; I have almost been expecting something to happen. When I came in I said to Maura [the ward sister], 'If I go too far, tell me' but she hasn't. I'm expecting someone to set limits and I don't know who is going to do it."

As we talked on, Rosalinda spoke of a trip she had made home the previous day. On the way she had stopped to get some food at the delicatessen where she often shopped. The son of the shop owner came out to the car with the food and as Rosalinda rooted through her bag for money he had got wet in the rain. Later, when she had phoned through to the shop with another order, the shop owner had been angry for

---

[14] J. H. Brodkey, "Passage Into Non-existence," *Independent on Sunday Magazine,* London, UK, 11 February (1996): 10-11.

keeping his son waiting in the rain and told her to have her money ready
in future. She had been shocked by this and felt "down" and "deflated"
afterwards. Once again she returned to old themes, speaking about her
mother and saying that she hoped that when she met her again she would
be as she was before she died and not "the horrible woman she was so
often before." She continued:

> "Mamma seemed to lose her fear of death, whereas I seem to be
> getting more frightened. … Maura was telling me that some people
> want to die alone. I don't. I want lots of people with me."

> "Have you seen anyone die?"

> "Yes, lots. Mamma used to get us out of bed in Sligo when someone
> was dying on the ward and bring us, my sister, brother and me,
> along to the bedside. 'This is what life's all about,' she'd say and
> get us to kneel at the bedside while the priest said the rosary. But I
> keep coming back to wondering what happens afterwards. I hate
> the idea of coming back as a fly or looking for an empty womb. …
> I've ordered a book on the world's great religions … "

> "Rosalinda, do you remember how I said at our last meeting that
> the feelings you have had in recent months of joy, hope,
> happiness—that these were not some illusion?"

> "And not side-effects of the morphine. I find that comforting."

> "Well, perhaps the 'ship of death' is not so much built of ideas,
> which can be read in books or what anyone else can say to you, as
> from the kind of experiences you have been living in recent months.
> Perhaps what you *can* do is to choose to trust in these experiences,
> even if there's no proof."

As I looked around her beautifully decorated room we began to speak
about her planned trip home over the holidays. I asked her how she was
feeling about the coming week and she replied "apprehensive" and began
discussing many of the practical details. She was planning to go out on
Christmas Eve and return on the evening of the twenty-sixth of
December. Sabha and Noel would be there to care for her and a nurse
would call in each morning. She asked about taking the special mattress
on her bed home with her and I reassured her that this would be possible.

> "It's getting better and better," she quipped.

> "Maybe you can trust that one too!" I returned.

7 January

The Christmas break had given me time to think about my work with Rosalinda. I had realized from my disappointment on receiving a gift of a book token from her that I had been unconsciously hoping she might have bought me a "ship of death" from Clodagh Redden's exhibition. I felt very ashamed to admit this to myself (as I do to write it here!), but it helped me to realize that even if we had become friends in our work together, I remained Rosalinda's "doctor" and she my "patient." Instead of inscribing the book token, she had included the following joke on a page torn from some book:

> An elderly man in hospital was overheard to say:
>
> "I'm not afraid to die ... dying isn't so bad ... the trouble is that you're so bloody stiff the next day."

With this Rosalinda helped me to refind my professional position in the nicest possible way.

When we met, Rosalinda spoke about how she had got on over Christmas. Instead of staying at home she had returned to sleep in her room in the palliative care unit each night and this seemed to have worked well. Since Christmas she had been "tired and sore." She put the soreness down to "all the pulling in and out of taxis" and felt that the tiredness was part of a post-Christmas anti-climax.

> "Before Christmas I was on a sort of high, the TV programme, all the talk of dying—but now I don't want to die and I'm frightened I'll be really sick. Do these new pains in my shoulder and leg mean the cancer is spreading? Have I got long? Will I be in pain? Will the drugs wear off? I feel I'm going to be an emotional mess ... I thought I'd let go of stuff from the past but it's got tentacles; the 'myth of analysis' that you can ever "get over" your painful past!"

Rosalinda's questions and distress reminded me of how she had been in the early weeks after admission.

> "No, Rosalinda, the new pain you have doesn't necessarily mean that the 'cancer is spreading,' although I can't be certain that this isn't the case. Perhaps one thing we should consider is doing another bone scan; it's the start of the New Year and it would help clarify what the situation is. Secondly, as you have discovered, palliative care can't promise 'no pain' but it can promise to be with you when you hurt and to do something about it, something that works and will go on working. And you're right; it is deeply disappointing

when we find ourselves back to square one in our emotional lives.
I think you're right in what you say about 'the myth of analysis' if
it creates the expectation that we can leave our past behind us. We
can't. We bring our past with us. The best we can hope for is to
learn to see things differently and to find a new and more creative
way of living with ourselves."

Previously we had discussed the idea of an "ethical will," the Jewish
concept of leaving behind something of the values, memories, and ideas
that had given one's life meaning and purpose. Rosalinda now came back
to this idea and said that she was determined to renew work on a set of tape
recordings she had started for Sabha. These, she hoped, would help fill in
some of the lesser known parts of her story for her daughter; details, for
example, of her early life growing up in Sligo and stories about her husband
and Sabha's father, Nathan, and their time together in the United States.

I said to Rosalinda that while I would be delighted for us to continue
working in this way together, perhaps she should consider whether she
still wanted to or if she might find it helpful to give it a break for a while.
I suggested she might like to think about this. Rosalinda immediately
replied that she wished to continue meeting, adding that it helped her
to look at what she needed to look at.

14 JANUARY

I was aware that Rosalinda had been very low, physically and
emotionally, during the past week. She had had more pain and was
nauseated, probably because of constipation. She was also anxious about
her bone scan, which was scheduled for the following day and she was
very much missing Sabha, who was on a trip to America. She said:

"I think it's definitely a case of post-Christmas depression ... it's
like how I've felt in the past when I was depressed but this time
I'm trapped. In the past I could distract myself, now I'm stuck with
it—I can't even read."

When Rosalinda said that she had not had any dreams, I suggested
that she might like to do some imagework, to "help her to tune in." She
was happy with this suggestion.

"Close your eyes and allow your breath to take you deep inside. ...
Imagine yourself in a favourite place in nature, somewhere familiar,
somewhere you love, somewhere special to you. Just be in this place.
Notice how you feel to be there. Now become aware that there is

another person in this place, someone who cares deeply about you, someone who knows your situation very well, someone wise, someone you trust, someone who understands you, someone you can be yourself with. Notice how you feel to be with this person. If it feels right, speak with this person. Tell her or him what you want to, ask a question if you will, put into words what it is you need. Be aware of how this person responds. ... Begin to prepare to leave, to say goodbye for now and when you are ready, return to the here and now."

Without opening her eyes, Rosalinda began to speak:

"It was Nathan. Before, I've felt I couldn't contact him. He was already occupied with his first wife, who also died of cancer. But this time he was there ... available ... with me. We were in our garden in New England, standing by the rocks that go into the sea at the end of the garden—it's where Eliot wrote 'The Dry Salvages.' It was sunny warm, early summer."

"Did you get a sense of what it was you wanted to say to him?"

As Rosalinda began to weep, she said:

"That I'm terrified ... that death is a gaping black hole ... that I sometimes fool myself that it's just like closing my eyes and going to sleep but it's not."

"And did you get a sense of how he might respond?"

"Well, it's nice to think that he might be there."

"Maybe that's all we can hope for ... it seems like there's nothing definite at this stage."

"How do others die; does their faith help them?"

"Some people with a strong religious faith are supported by it; a lot of people don't look at it; they carry on as if it's not happening— that's what's different about you; you're looking at it straight in the face. Right now you seem to be *in* that black hole. Do you know those lines of the Welsh poet R. S. Thomas?

> It is too late to start
> For destinations not of the heart.
> I must stay here with my hurt.[15]

---

[15] R. S. Thomas, *Collected Poems 1945-1990* (London, UK: Phoenix Giants, 1993), p. 120.

Smiling through her tears, Rosalinda said:

> "Thank you for that. … It helps to put it into words."

17 January

The bone scan result showed extensive progression in Rosalinda's bone secondaries. In addition to deterioration of the known deposit in her neck, there were several new "hot spots," most notably in her pelvis. By the time I went to talk to her about this, she had already had conversations with others on the team and knew the results. I confirmed that, although there had been some deterioration, "things weren't that bad" and that we would be continuing on with the same treatments as before. Rosalinda was tired and wanting to sleep. She said how glad she was that Sabha had returned safely.

21 January

Rosalinda had celebrated her sixty-sixth birthday a couple of days previously. That evening she had been out to dinner with Sabha and the previous day had a party with all the nurses on the ward. In general she was in good form and physically stronger and more comfortable than she had been. Earlier I had spoken with Deirdre who told me that Rosalinda was using their sessions together to work on her tapes for Sabha. Rosalinda greeted me by telling me how sleepy she was, adding:

> "I expect this is the beginning of the end. … If I just doze off, that's OK … but I'm not quite ready. … I still have some work to do."

I asked her about this and she talked of the tapes she was working on for Sabha. I also explained that there were a number of other possible explanations for her increased levels of drowsiness, in particular the fact that she had recently been started on new anticonvulsant medication for her pain, which could be causing some sedation. She replied:

> "Oh good! Can we reduce that, and can we please do some visualization?"

> "Of course we can. Was there anything in particular you wanted to look at?"

> "I was just talking with Angela [the social worker]. I asked her what she believed about life after death and if belief made a difference in people she knew. She said she had a strong faith … didn't say in what but I presume in life continuing in some way."

I suggested that we proceed with the imagework and see where this brought her:

> "Close your eyes and bring your attention to your breathing. Be aware of this rhythm of receiving and letting go ... receiving what is needed for life in this moment and letting go what needs to be let go of ... and as you continue to breathe be aware of your body, of how you feel in your body at the moment ... this body, which holds you, which connects you to the ground, to the earth. Now, begin to imagine yourself in nature in a place that is special to you ... be in this place, notice it, open to the experience of being there. Know that you are going to meet with a wise being—this may be a person, or it may be an animal or it may be an object. Consider what you would like to ask such a being if you had the opportunity ... perhaps it would be a question such as you put to Angela ... maybe it's a question, maybe it's a request. As you get a clearer sense of this, you become aware that this wise being is nearby—notice, observe, be aware of how it is to be with this being. Find a way of greeting this being. Find a way of asking your question or making your request. Notice ... listen to the response. Know that you will be leaving this wise being and this place shortly. Find a way of saying farewell. Gradually begin to come back to the here and now and when you are ready, open your eyes."

Rosalinda had fallen asleep. About ten minutes later she opened her eyes and said, looking across at her clock on the bedside table: "I've been asleep."

"Yes you have ... do you recall anything from the visualization?"

"No, but there was a nice feeling ... something pleasant ... " [By now Rosalinda's eyes had closed again and she was almost muttering, as if on the edge of sleep] "I was in Australia ... something about eucalyptus trees ... they're such beautiful trees; native to Australia but transported to the Indian desert in an attempt to preserve water in the land and prevent the desert spreading but it had the opposite effect. They drank all the water and dried out the land even more. A grove of eucalyptus, they look so beautiful ... by a river ... yet they are somehow stunted ... they are not able to grow fully because there is not enough water ... maybe some will be OK but some won't. We shouldn't tamper with nature. Something about Mamma in there also. I wish I could trust her, believe her ... her last words to me were something about me being her most special child. But it's hard to forget that she pulled me back and down so many times."

"What kind of response do you imagine you might get were you to ask your mother a question like you asked Angela?"

"She seemed to find peace close to the end—she had a very legalistic belief, which wasn't much comfort to her during her life, but she did seem to find peace. ... I wish I could be open to this."

"And Australia?"

"I've never been there."

"Eucalyptus trees?"

"I love them—such slender, beautiful trees ... I love their leaves in bouquets. Some varieties have leaves that are scythe-shaped, a pale mauve colour, beautiful in the wind ... that's something I'd love to do ... donate some trees to the hospice; maybe some eucalyptus or maybe silver birch. I have eucalyptus in my garden front and back and silver birch against a hedge of evergreen ... their *white* bark ... yes, maybe a grove of silver birch ... that's something I'd have loved to do: plant lots of silver birch around my house, loosely ... to let the light in. Yes, a house in a grove of trees, letting in dappled light and some climbers growing up through them ... and a stream ... maybe that's what heaven will be like. ... I hope so."

"You talk of trees with love."

"Yes, I love trees ... then someone explained that they were phallic symbols."

"That's a very limited view. Trees are metaphors for more than that."

"Yes, I suppose life itself ... 'the Tree of Life.'"

"Trees just seem to be there, they don't have to *do* anything to prove themselves, they blossom in who and what they are. 'Lungs of the world'—breathing in as we breathe out, breathing out as we breathe in. As much in the dark underground as in the light above ... silently interconnecting with our lives."

"Yes, I'd love to donate a grove of birch trees. ... It would be wonderful to see them in before spring arrives."

By now Rosalinda was animated and fully awake. I told her of my meeting at traffic lights that morning with the so-called "Eco-warriors," a group of people who were living rough in a forest under threat to protect it from developers. And I told her of a man I was caring for whose dying desire was to have his small plot of forest replanted with deciduous trees. The hour was up. She commented:

"At least the focus wasn't all on *me* and my process this time."

It felt to me as if the imagework in this session had crossed into dreamtime. Maybe this is why we were in Australia for no obvious reason?

The tree that emerged as "wise being" brought with it a mix of opposite and ambivalent images; desert and water, stunting and growth. The fact that the grove of trees was next to a river was reminiscent of the earlier imagework meeting with Kate by the water's edge. And there was the presence of Rosalinda's mother also holding opposite and ambivalent associations; the one who blessed her as "special" and the one who held back and stunted her growth, the one with a dry, "legalistic" religious belief in life and the one who found "peace," and moisture, at the edge of the unknown. While acknowledging the danger of romanticizing what was happening here and while accepting the risk of wishful thinking in Rosalinda's vision of what "heaven" might be like, the presence of the tree as "wise being" seemed to include these complex and contradictory shades in a bigger picture. Was this also what Rosalinda was articulating in her desire to see a grove of trees established and growing in this place of dying?

28 JANUARY

Rosalinda had developed pneumonia and heart failure during the night of the twenty-first of January. She was very ill at that time and, despite active treatment, it looked as if she might die. Sabha was constantly at her bedside. When I had called in to see her on the morning of the twenty-third it was obvious she was beginning to improve. She was sipping white wine through a straw as Sabha helped her with her meal. "I love being fed by Sabha," she had said. The following weekend she had discussions with the duty-doctor about her antibiotics. She had asked if she would die without them. When told that she might, she asked if she could think about this. The feeling on ward rounds on the twenty-sixth was that although her condition had stabilized, it now looked as if she was very much in the terminal phase of her illness and that she would most likely die quite soon. There was a feeling of sadness among the team, but there was also a sense that Rosalinda herself was "serene" and that she may be ready to "slip away."

When I called in to see her on the morning of the twenty-eighth, she was heavy-eyed and extremely drowsy. At first she was somewhat bothered, since she had been expecting to be visited by a doctor she had met at the previous hospital. She also had concerns about her finances and how these would cover her long stay in hospital. I attempted to reassure her on these matters and asked her how she was feeling after the past week's events. As she began to speak, it was clear that her recall of recent events was patchy. She spoke movingly of being cared for by Sabha, adding, "She's such a gentle creature." When I reminded her of what she had said to me about being fed by Sabha, she laughed and said:

> "I remember waking and seeing Sabha sitting there in the dark and wondering should I let go and slip away. Could I? Could she?"

When I reminded Rosalinda of her questions about the antibiotics, she did not remember but it was evident that this was not now of concern to her. She asked:

> "Will I know if something like this happens again that I'm dying? And what will it be like?"
>
> "You have spoken of how gentle and easy and peaceful these last few days have been; well, it will probably be something like that. A gradual slowing down of your body and then slipping into a deep sleep."

I then asked:

> "Do you recall any dreams in all this?"
>
> "Flowers ... paddocks of flowers ... all colours ... "
>
> "Do you remember the eucalyptus trees of last week and the grove of silver birch?"
>
> "No."

Following our previous session I had read over two poems I had been reminded of. I had brought these in with me and I now offered to read them to Rosalinda. She said she would like that.

> "The first of these is called 'Lost' by the American poet David Wagoner. It is could be seen as a reply to the question, 'What do I do when I am lost in the forest?'
>
> > Stand still. The trees ahead and the bushes beside you
> > Are not lost. Wherever you are is called Here,
> > And you must treat it as a powerful stranger,
> > Must ask permission to know it and be known.
> > The forest breathes. Listen. It answers,
> > I have made this place around you.
> > If you leave it, you may come back again, saying Here.
> > No two trees are the same to Raven.
> > No two branches are the same to Wren.
> > If what a tree of bush does is lost to you,

> You are surely lost. Stand still. The forest knows
> Where you are. You must let it find you.[16]

As I finished this, Rosalinda asked me to reread it and then to read it again. We then sat in silence for some time. Then I introduced the second poem:

"This one was written by Rainer Maria Rilke. It's called 'Autumn':

> The leaves are falling, falling as from far,
> as though above were withering farthest gardens;
> they fall with a denying attitude.
> And night by night, down into solitude,
> the heavy earth falls far from every star.
> We are all falling. This hand's falling too—
> all have this falling-sickness none withstands.
> And yet there's One whose gently-holding hands
> this universal falling can't fall through.[17]

Once again, Rosalinda wanted me to reread this poem several times and especially the last two lines until she had learnt them for herself. "Whose hands we can't fall through ... Yes, that's what I want," she said, laughing quietly to herself. She then asked me to place the copies of the poems I had brought for her in Jung's *Man and his Symbols,* which was sitting on a nearby table. "I had thought I'd do all this reading," she said, pointing to a stack of books on the side-table, including her newly acquired copy of *Great Religions of the* World.

"Instead, you're living it," I commented.

"Thank you," she nodded; "that's putting it nicely."

4 FEBRUARY

Rosalinda's condition had remained weak but stable since the previous week. On the third of February she had become chesty, despite still being on antibiotics and diuretics. Overnight she had a severe bout of neck pain and needed a lot of additional analgesia to get her comfortable. The nurses were distressed and some felt that we should

---

[16] David Wagoner, *Who Shall be the Sun?* (Bloomington: Indiana University Press, 1978), p. 5.

[17] Rainer Maria Rilke, *Selected Poems,* trans. J. B. Leishman (London, UK: Penguin, 1964), p. 25.

increase her medication significantly to make a repeat of this impossible, even if this meant increasing her level of sedation. During the previous week I had wondered at times if we were accurate in our reading of recent events and had begun to think that perhaps Rosalinda might pull through on this occasion. I now realized that this was not the case. The nurses told me that when Rosalinda was awake earlier in the morning she had said to them that she was unsure whether or not to see me that afternoon but had then decided she would. I felt somewhat hurt by this. I was also reminded of my feelings at Christmas time and wondered if it was now time to move more into the background.

When I called in, Rosalinda was deeply asleep. I called her name and touched her hand but was unable to wake her. I sat with her for fifteen minutes or so and then left. Outside Sabha was waiting to speak with me. We talked about what was happening. I said I felt the end was very close. It was evident that Sabha was aware of this. I told her that Rosalinda had wondered at our last meeting if she [Sabha] was ready to "let go." She replied, "When is one ever ready for something like this?"

5 FEBRUARY

On rounds the following day I heard that Rosalinda had been settled in the early part of the night but had then become confused and agitated in the early hours of the morning. She had pulled out her portable syringe driver and wandered out of her room. The nurse on duty had brought her back to bed and the duty doctor had come in to reassess her. She was given some additional sedation, started back on her syringe pump and she soon went back to sleep.

When I went into Rosalinda's room, her brother was sitting with her. As he left, Sabha and Noel came in. Rosalinda was drowsy but lucid, as though she was on the edge of her dreams, and this quality wove in and out of her conversation. She said:

> "Tomorrow's the sixth of February. That's Mamma anniversary and my wedding anniversary. I'd like to die tomorrow: three in one … "

> "And have you any pain, Rosalinda?"

> "No."

> "Frightened?"

"No. ... But I'd like to make a speech. ... I want to thank you all ... I've sorted out with Sabha what I want done afterwards. ... Now, all out! I'd like to talk to Dr. Kearney on his own ... "

Turning to me she said:

"I want to thank you for everything you have done for me."

"Thank *you*, Rosalinda. ... I hope you find yourself moving into a place of peace and beauty. I'm thinking of those beautiful trees you spoke about a couple of weeks ago ... "

"Yes, that's something that I want to do. I want to plant that grove of trees. Pass me that book, it has the name of a landscape gardener who could do the job. Yes, those white and silver boughs ... winter is so long ... "

"How about if I speak with Sabha about this? She will take care of it and we will do what we can to help her. I too would love to see those trees out there."

"Perhaps I can't do it all. ... I want to thank you. I wish you well."

"Thank you, Rosalinda, it's been lovely to know you and to work with you and I too wish you well."

I had been sitting facing the same way as she was, my hand resting on her arm. I rose and took her hand when saying goodbye. I felt like kissing her. Instead I shook her hand. Outside I spoke with Sabha.

Rosalinda died very peacefully on the tenth of February. When awake during those final days she was in no pain. Sabha was constantly with her and her room was always full with family and close friends. The sadness of that time was infused with celebration. Tears and champagne, Rosalinda at the centre.

CHAPTER TWELVE

Bill

A surgeon colleague asked me to see Bill for "terminal care." Six months previously he had performed a laparotomy on this seventy-year-old man and found that his newly diagnosed pancreatic cancer was inoperable. Not only was the tumor too large to remove, but there were extensive liver secondaries. He had told Bill the diagnosis and had promised him that he would help him if problems arose in the future.

As Bill sat beside his bed I could see that his legs were as swollen as tree trunks. The contrast was stark with his gaunt torso and spindly arms. He had a high facial colour, more suggestive of someone who has worked out of doors for many years than of the civil servant he was. He sat hunched slightly forward with lively eyes and a slight smile as I explained who I was and how I hoped I could help him.

Well, Bill told me, if that is what I did, he was not really sure I could be of much help to him. He was not really bothered by pain. Yes, his appetite was poor and he was "weak as water" but these did not bother him much either. One thing I might do, he added, was to tell him exactly what was going on because he had things he needed to sort out. I responded by asking him what he already understood of his situation.

"That I have cancer in my pancreas, which has spread to my liver."

"That's what I understand as well. And to judge from how it's been for you in recent times and those swollen legs and from looking at your blood results, it looks as if this is continuing to progress."

"Will I get home again?"

"What are your home circumstances?"

"I have my own home. I live on my own. I have two sisters living in Dublin. They're both as helpful as they can be."

"At the moment you say you're so weak you need two nurses to help you walk a few steps to the bathroom. I can arrange physiotherapy for you and prescribe some medications to try to boost your energy and help you lose some of that fluid from your legs, but it's impossible to say at the moment what kind of progress you'll make. We'll have to wait and see."

"It doesn't look good then, does it?"

"Not great, I'm sorry to say. ... You mentioned you had things you needed to do; do you mind me asking what these are? I'm wondering if there's anything I can do to help here?"

"I don't think so. ... It's to do with a small patch of forest I own in Wicklow. I bought it a number of years ago from Coillte [the Irish Forestry Board]. It's a small thin strip of land on the opposite side of the road to a large Coillte forest. They didn't want it, a bit awkward I suppose, so they sold it off. I have been down there every few weeks to see it over the years. I've watched the Douglas firs grow into massive trees. Nine months ago I had some of the trees cut down and sold the wood; about a quarter of the total area. Now I want to replant that area with broad-leaved trees. I was on to Coillte the other day but the man I spoke with more or less told to me not to bother them."

As Bill spoke, his voice was noticeably more animated and stronger than it had been. I felt very moved by his determination to care for his forest in this way. It seemed really important that he continue to work to bring this to completion. I asked him about Douglas firs and what types of broad-leaved trees he had in mind for replanting. He replied, "beech and oak." I suggested he should try to contact Coillte again. Perhaps he would get through to someone more helpful this time. Meanwhile we could start the treatments I had mentioned and see how things went. I told him I would be back to see him again soon. My hope as I left him was that he would still have enough time to do what he needed to do.

I called back to see Bill a few days later. In the interim I had read about the Douglas fir, the *Pseudotsuga meniesii*,[1] and learnt that:

---

[1] *Field Guide to the Trees and Shrubs of Britain* (London, UK: Reader's Digest, 1981), p. 218.

> This very tall, conical tree grows to 180 feet (55 m) in Britain and
> 325 feet (100 m) in its native North American Rocky Mountains.
> [The bark] is dark grey or purple with age; fissured and corky. After
> the coastal redwoods, the Douglas fir is the tallest tree growing on
> the North American West Coast. This magnificent conifer is named
> after David Douglas, the plant collector who introduced its seeds
> to Britain in 1827. The newcomer was widely planted at first as a
> decorative tree, particularly in the policies, or private woodlands,
> around Scottish mansions. Many of Britain's Douglas firs are not
> yet old enough to produce the first-class timber of North America,
> where it is called the Oregon pine.

As I entered Bill's room he was snoozing in the chair by his bed. I
was struck by how emaciated he looked. His grotesquely enormous legs
again underlined his frailty. He awoke with a smile as I called his name.
Telling me that there had not been any significant improvement yet in
either his energy or leg swelling on the new medication, he added that
he was really too weak to co-operate with the physiotherapist. In terms
of the agreed plan to try and improve his mobility, the nurses had been
encouraging him to do more for himself but this was only emphasizing
his limitations and proving counterproductive. We agreed to a change
in strategy. While continuing the new medications over the coming
weekend to give them a final trial, we would all take a gentler line with
his mobilization. Bill also complained of a new symptom; a feeling of
"aching pressure" just below his right ribs. Having palpated his abdomen,
I prescribed some analgesia for this discomfort, which was being caused
by liver capsular swelling, yet further evidence of his steadily deteriorating
condition. He interrupted my thoughts by saying:

> "I got through to a different man in Coillte. He was really interested
> and is going to send me out a map so I can give him all the details."

It was obvious that he was delighted by this.

I next called back about four days later. Bill was sitting by a table in
his room working on some papers. He had been painstakingly coloring
in different parts of an Ordnance Survey map he had just received from
his contact in Coillte. On a smaller scale map of the area he showed me
his little strip of forest, on a hillside not far outside the town of Aughrim.
On the other map he explained that the upper quarter, crossed with red
diagonal lines, was the area of cut forest where he wanted the replanting
done. The lower three-quarters of the strip, partially coloured in with

green lines, was the remaining area of mature Douglas firs. As he
continued to colour in the map, he bent forward in concentration over
the table. He said:

> "I know a number of people who would love to get their hands on
> that land—speculators. But it's really important to me that it's
> replanted. And I want broad-leaved trees this time, oak and beech.
> … I discussed this with my friend in Coillte … he seemed to
> understand. I feel he will follow through with this and I've spoken
> to my sister about this also. She knows my wishes."

I watched Bill in his concentrated effort as he spoke. It was now clear
to me that the treatments had not worked and that his prognosis was very
short, perhaps a week or so at the most. This was likely to be among his
final acts. I felt there was something heroic, courageous, and generous
in what he was doing.

When I called to see Bill three days later he was beginning to die.
The previous day his condition had suddenly deteriorated. He had no
pain but had become extremely weak. Since then he had been sleeping
most of the time. One of his sisters was sitting by his bed as I entered his
room. Bill was lying, curled up on his side, asleep in his bed. After a little
while he opened a single eye to me.

> "Hello," I said, "did you manage to get that letter off about your
> trees?"
>
> "Yes," he smiled, both eyes now open, "a great achievement."
>
> "A great achievement," I echoed.

I could see he was comfortable and he seemed at peace. I said:

> "Bill, in a few days time I will be traveling near Aughrim. I will
> take time to try and find your forest. I would love to see it. …
> Goodbye for now."

Outside I spoke with his sister and told her that time was now very
short.

> "I'm glad he sorted out his business with the forest," she said. "It
> was important for him. He can rest easy now."

That morning as I was driving to work I had met the "Eco-warriors"
distributing information on their campaign to save trees in a broad-leafed
forest not far from Bill's plantation in County Wicklow. That afternoon

I had shared his story with Rosalinda when she spoke of her desire to plant a grove of silver birches in the hospice. That evening I had heard from a friend, who told me of forty great trees, which had been felled on their lands in a recent storm. That night Bill died. Threads in a pattern bigger than each of us and not of our making. A dreaming of trees or the trees' dreaming?

Conclusion

At the beginning of this book I suggested that we should ask ourselves what we regard as the fundamental responsibility of healthcare. Do we see this only in terms of intervening to treat our patients' pain, or do we also understand it in terms of working with patients in their suffering? My thesis throughout has been that healthcare has a dual responsibility to patients in their pain and their suffering because, whether we like it or not, the experience of illness includes both. Patients need both a surface *and* a deep, a classical *and a* quantum, a Hippocratic *and* an Asklepian approach to them in their illness.

In the last chapter I told the story of Bill. Although the beauty of this tale lies in its simplicity, I am aware in telling it of a danger of sounding naïve, or romantic, or both. "This is all very nice—but it never seems to happen like this with my patients," I can hear the battle-weary clinician mutter dismissively. With this in mind I want to share one final story before ending. I do this in acknowledgement of the fact that even when we consciously attempt to offer our patients an integrated clinical approach, one which combines the best of both Hippocratic medicine and Asklepian healing, it does not mean that things will always work out the way we would like them to. Such patients remind us that we have hardly begun to understand the phenomena of human suffering and healing, and challenge us to continue in this quest.

Mary's Story

Mary was in her early fifties and had advanced intra-abdominal spread from a primary cancer of the bowel. She was widowed and had three children, two daughters and a son, all in their early twenties, who were living and working from home. For some weeks the palliative home care team had been visiting her at home. She was extremely weak and wasted, with some mild discomfort from the malignant involvement of her liver, but this responded well to analgesia and she soon became physically very comfortable. At the first home care visit Mary spoke of how she was "terrified of dying." She had heard how palliative care was as concerned with patients' "inner experience" as with their bodily symptoms and this is where she particularly wanted help. The social worker from the home care team had begun to visit Mary at home and had several conversations with her about her fears and concerns. Many of these centred on the almost unbearable emotional pain she experienced when she thought of leaving her children, and in particular her son, who was her youngest child and to whom she felt especially close.

At the next meeting with the social worker, Mary announced that she wanted to be admitted to the inpatient palliative care unit to continue "to prepare for death." Despite contrary advice from her family doctor and the home care team and reassurance from her children that they wanted her to stay at home, Mary continued to insist on admission. This was then arranged on what was hoped would be a temporary, respite basis.

Mary was admitted to the palliative care unit shortly after this and remained there until her death some ten weeks later. During this time she was not troubled by physical symptoms but her emotional pain and suffering seemed to intensify with each passing day. She had worked with a cancer support group as a counselor before her own illness and so was very familiar with approaches such as visualization, art therapy, and massage. She enrolled in each of these programmes within the palliative care unit and her day was filled with the various therapy sessions to the extent that her family, as well as the nursing and medical staff, had some difficulty in finding times to visit. Meanwhile, the same social worker as before continued to work with her and her family.

At this stage a case conference was held to discuss the situation. Everyone agreed that Mary was in great distress, and various carers and therapists reported a similar tale of how their time together appeared to be of no real consolation to her. Each told of how Mary used their meeting to talk about the same issues over and over again, without any real sense of movement, their discussion seeming to bring neither resolution nor deepening, rather a feeling of going around in the same small circle of anguish and despair. There was broad agreement that approaches which enabled Mary to feel "held" and connected to objective reality, in particular working with the body through massage and the nursing and medical aspects of care, were more likely to be of benefit than either "talking therapies" or "depth work" at this stage. The ward sister proposed a simplified care plan to Mary, who seemed content and somewhat relieved with this, as were her family.

Over the following days there was little change in Mary's situation. She continued to be frightened, agitated, and distressed. By then it was also apparent that she was physically much weaker and that her prognosis was probably very short, perhaps a week or two at the most. Different members of the caring team reassured her family that by continuing to care for Mary in this way, she should come to an easier place in herself. Sadly, this did not happen. On the contrary, each day seemed to bring Mary into new dimensions of anguish. The only relief she appeared to have came when she was asleep. When she was awake, she wanted someone with her constantly and even then was demanding and restless and beyond all efforts to bring her consolation.

Mary was already on some regular anxiolytic medication. At a team meeting held at this stage, a decision was made to increase her sedation in a further effort to lessen her emotional and psychological distress. Her family agreed with this. During the following days, Mary slept for long periods. On some occasions when awake she appeared calm and at ease with her family but at other times she again became restless and agitated. She was by then very frail and it was evident that she was beginning to die. She remained asleep during her final forty-eight hours, with her family at her bedside. They said they had found the previous weeks "harrowing" but that those last days were "a comfort," and that they could be with her more easily. They were all at her bedside when she died.

SOME REFLECTIONS IN LIGHT OF MARY'S STORY

Mary's is not a story with a happy ending. Despite her own considerable efforts, and those of her carers, she had an extremely difficult time in her dying. Her story illustrates both the value and the limitations of the Hippocratic and Asklepian models in the presence of intractable human suffering. While it proved impossible to relieve Mary's suffering, it was possible, to some extent at least, to contain and lessen her distress through a combination of both these approaches.

"To Care and Not to Care"

Although Mary's physical pain had been an issue at an earlier stage, it was her psychological and existential suffering that dominated her final weeks. Those who cared for her did not question whether or not this suffering was part of their clinical responsibility. As the source of her overwhelming distress this was their primary concern as they did their best to help her. One question that might be asked in this context, however, is whether or not the responsibilities of carers to those who suffer can or should be qualified in any way? Are there, in other words, limits to the responsibilities of carers to those who suffer?

I believe there are. I also believe, however, that these are not so much determined by that person's history ("this is a lifetime's worth of emotional, psychological, and existential distress and therefore not really our concern"); nor by logistical, financial, ethical, or philosophical considerations, as by the intrinsic nature of suffering itself. Although the carer can feel deeply for, share in, and, indeed, agonize with another in his or her suffering, in some fundamental way, *the suffering belongs to that person,* and it is *only* that individual who can live with and through this experience.

Psychiatrist Averil Stedeford suggests that:

> When we are with a patient [who is in suffering and dying] we should never lose sight of the fact that it is their own death that they are facing and no one else can do this for them.[1]

On the same theme, medical ethicist Daniel Callahan writes:

> What life itself may give us at its end is a death that seems, in the suffering it brings, to make no sense. That is a *terrible* problem, but it is the patient's problem and not the doctor's. The doctor can relieve pain if it is present, make the patient as comfortable as possible, and be another human presence. Otherwise, the patient must do it on her own. We have no resource left but ourselves at that point.[2]

At first glance these words may sound callous or, indeed, uncaring and be misunderstood as a recipe for calculated indifference to patients in their suffering. This is not the case. There are occasions where we are unable to help another in suffering because we do not know how or

---

[1] Averil Stedeford, "Hospice: A Safe Place to Suffer?" *Palliative Medicine* 1 (1987): 74.

[2] Daniel Callahan, *The Troubled Dream of Life* (New York: Touchstone, 1993), p. 102.

because we have come to the limits of our expertise, and know of no other intervention that may help. Our responsibility here is to do all we can to find this expertise, if it exists, elsewhere and to make it available to the patient. There are other occasions where we have also done all this and concluded that, unfortunately, no such additional expertise exists, and no further intervention is possible. This is where we need to pause in our efforts and make a mental switch in our way of thinking about suffering. We may now be at that place where, as author C. S. Lewis puts it when writing of his own experience of grief, we have to accept that, "There is nothing to do with suffering except to suffer it,"[3] to which we might add, *"and only the bereaved person him- or herself can do this."*

It is not so much a question, therefore, of the carer's responsibility to the one who suffers ending here, as of both parties now moving together into a new situation of shared responsibility. The carer's part is to stay with and hold that person in his or her suffering; the patient's is to live with and hopefully through that suffering, as only he or she can. The inner stance this demands of the carer is well described by the poet T.S. Eliot in the following extract from his poem *Ash Wednesday:*

> Teach us to care and not to care
> Teach us to sit still
> Even among these rocks,
> Our peace in His will
> And even among these rocks
> Sister, mother
> And spirit of the river, spirit of the sea,
> Suffer me not to be separated
>
> And let my cry come unto Thee.[4]

"To care" speaks of our responsibility to the one who suffers. "Not to care" points to the limits in that responsibility, as we acknowledge that some of the responsibility in suffering belongs to the one who suffers. "To care" for the patient who suffers means doing all we can to lessen his or her distress and staying with that person when there is nothing left to do. "Not to care" means trusting that "even among [the] rocks" of impotence, helplessness, meaninglessness, and despair, some deeper wisdom within that person's psyche can respond to his or her silent cry.

---

[3] C. S. Lewis, *A Grief Observed* (London, UK: Faber & Faber, 1961), p. 29.
[4] T. S. Eliot, *Collected Poems 1909-1962* (London, UK: Faber & Faber), p. 105.

The Containment of Suffering

The therapeutic use of self by carers is as important as the knowledge and skills they bring to their professional role, and of primary importance when it comes to being with another in suffering. We have already noted how this involves communicating, encouraging, and, especially, *containing.* "Containing" means psychologically holding the one who suffers even when there is nothing left to do, and no matter what happens. It means recognizing that attending to, thinking about, and working with one's own reactions as a carer facilitates the process of psychological and spiritual healing in the other. The containment of suffering validates the humanity of the patient and the wisdom of his or her own psyche.

Containment was all those caring for Mary had to offer her in the final stages of her illness and it demanded a significant personal involvement by each member of the team. Those who cared for Mary were aware of their containing role. They knew that they were dealing with suffering, which, although they too experienced it, was primarily hers rather than theirs, and they were all trying, in spite of all they saw and felt to the contrary, to trust her own psyche's way in this. In the process of containing Mary in her suffering, her carers lived with feelings of sadness, disappointment, impotence, and guilt. They felt they had failed both her and her family's expectations of them, yet they also sensed that perhaps this was as good as it could possibly be in these particular circumstances. Afterwards, they were left with many questions.

- Had they interpreted the situation correctly, or had they missed something?
- Could things have been said or done differently and, if so, might it have worked out better for Mary?
- Had their understanding of their containing role been a rationalization to ease their own profound sense of failure?
- Was their eventual use of strong sedation more a palliation of their own suffering than of hers?

Such questions do not have easy answers. They remind us, however, that the actual process of the therapeutic use of self in the containment of suffering can be costly in emotional and psychological terms for the carer, and they highlight once again the need for "containment of the containers" through individual therapy and clinical supervision.

Working with the Healing Power of Nature

The basic premise of Asklepian healing is that there is within the psyche a spontaneous dynamic towards balance and wholeness. I have referred to this as the "healing power of nature" because it describes an integral part of our essential nature, which is, I believe, at one with the deeper rhythms of the natural world. Nature is neither sentimental nor romantic, yet there is within the natural realm a constant striving towards inclusion. Joy and suffering, illness and disease, life and death—each have a place within this bigger, broader ecology. I agree with cultural historian and theologian Thomas Berry when he says:

> [Although] it is composed of both constructive and destructive forces, it is ultimately a benign universe.[5]

To work with dreams is a way of working with nature. Although "dreamwork" can be seen in the literal sense of attending to dreams, we have also considered it as a metaphor for inner or soul-work, in whatever form this may take. This work may be through art, music, or the body. It may be through meditation. It may be through spending time in the natural world, whether this is working in one's garden or being in wilderness. It may be by engaging in what Kreinheder calls those "meaningful things done habitually, without a thought of their doing,"[6] or by participating in life as a waking dream.

In Mary's story, the "dreamwork" did not happen, as one might have expected it to, with her imagework or art therapy sessions. For her, inner work and outer work were one and the same thing. Here, dreamwork meant attending to what Callahan calls "the troubled dream"[7] of her everyday life. Here, care of the body and tender witnessing of all Mary lived was also care of the soul. With this, the locus of hope changed for the carers from the possibility of "making it all better" to that implicit in Saunders's phrase, "The way care is given can reach the most hidden places."[8]

---

[5] Thomas Berry, "The Sacred Universe," in *The Forsaken Garden,* ed. Nancy Ryley (Illinois: Quest Books, 1998), p. 246.
[6] Kreinheder (1991), p. 110.
[7] Callahan (1993).
[8] Cicely Saunders, Foreword, in Michael Kearney (1996), p. 12.

Dreamwork is not just another Hippocratic—albeit psychological—intervention, dependent for its "success" on the knowledge and skills of the carer. For some, such work may make things easier and lessen distress, but for others—at least in the short term—it may, as we have seen in many of the stories earlier in the book, have quite the opposite effect. Outcome is not the fundamental issue in dreamwork. What matters here is whether or not we trust the psyche. Are we willing and committed to working with nature in the service of wholeness, within the containment of relationship and effective treatment and care, *whatever* this may bring for patient—and carer?

TOWARDS MORE CONSCIOUS CARING

The unconscious workings of the psyche are an integral part of what happens in healthcare. This is a fact, whether we like it or not. The real question is how can we recognize and respond to such processes, for even a lack of response is itself a definite statement, which may be heard by the other as a dismissal of psyche, or, worse still, as something to be ashamed of.

My intention throughout has not been to encourage carers to dabble in what is outside their area of expertise but to suggest that all who care must know how to attend to unconscious as well as conscious events in others and in themselves in ways that are appropriate. This process of "conscious caring" takes many possible forms. In the clinical setting it may happen as we encourage a patient to talk about the dream that so disturbed the previous night's sleep, or as we listen to a patient who is sharing a significant memory that has just resurfaced, or as we silently contain within our own body and psyche another's unutterable distress. It also happens as we notice what we are feeling and how we are behaving in the presence of suffering. Occasionally it means acknowledging that we are out of our depth, professionally, or personally, or both, and that we need the help of someone more experienced in this area.

It is not possible to care consciously in this way unless we are committed to working with the unconscious in our personal and professional lives. This is why we must look to a closer alliance between the disciplines of healthcare and psychology. Healthcare needs to consider the relevance of the radical concepts and discoveries of psychodynamic theory, depth psychology, and ecopsychology and to ask the help of experts in these areas. Their advice is needed on how to translate these ideas into a language that is both accessible and acceptable, on how to design a broader and more inclusive system of healthcare education and on how to operate programmes of clinical supervision and reflective practice.

It would be naive, however, to think that such a change in the culture of healthcare could be a simple matter. Things are the way they are for two reasons:

- Firstly, because the healthcare system has worked and, for the most part, continues to work reasonably well this way.
- Secondly, because the existing set-up protects carers from what may be perceived as the threat of the unconscious.

Any plan to make caring more conscious needs to accommodate the fact that the status quo of contemporary healthcare involves institutionalized (and unconscious) defense systems against the unconscious. Change cannot happen here unless the benefits (as well as the limitations) of these defense systems are appreciated. Before change is possible, we have to acknowledge that these defenses are valuable and recognize how they play an important part in the success of contemporary healthcare. They explain how carers have been able to stay close to others in their suffering without being overwhelmed by it. They explain how carers have continued to care.

Although the challenge to find a more conscious form of caring is daunting, the first step in this process is both clear and accessible. As carers we must each begin to befriend our own unconscious. We shall then discover from experience that it is possible to trust the psyche, which is nature's voice within, and which can lead us through suffering to a place of greater wholeness.

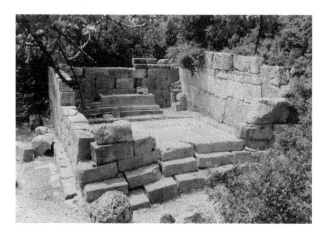

At Epidauros, in the stillness, in the great peace that came over me,
I heard the heart of the world beat. I know what the cure is: it is to
give up, to relinquish, to surrender, so that our little hearts may
beat in unison with the great heart of the world.

—Henry Miller[9]

[9] Henry Miller, *The Colossus of Maroussi* (New York: New Directions, 1958), p. 77.

Bibliography and Further Reading

Ahmedzai, Sam H. "Five Years: Five Threads," editorial, *Progress in Palliative Care* 5, 1997.

Aizenstat, Stephen. "Jungian Psychology and the World Unconscious," in *Ecopsychology; Restoring the Earth, Healing the Mind,* ed. T. Roszak, M.E. Gomes, and A. D. Kanner. Sierra Club Books, 1995.

Baylor, B. and Parnall, P. *The Other Way to Listen.* Atheneum, 1978.

Becker, Ernest. *The Denial of Death.* Free Press Paperbacks, 1973.

Berry, P. *Echo's Subtle Body.* Spring Publications, 1982.

Berry, Thomas. *The Dream of the Earth.* Sierra Club Books, 1988.

———. "The Sacred Universe," in *The Forsaken Garden,* ed. Nancy Ryley. Quest Books, 1998.

Bion, W.R. "A Theory of Thinking," *International Journal of Psycho-Analysis,* 43(4-5), 1962.

Boer, C., trans. *The Homeric Hymns.* Spring Publications, 1970.

Bonnivier, Joy Fest. "A Peer Supervision Group: Put Countertransference to Work," *Journal of Psychosocial Nursing* 30(5), 1992.

Bosnak, R. *A Little Course in Dreams.* Shambhala, 1986.

———. *Dreaming with an AIDS Patient.* Shambhala, 1989.

———. *Tracks in the Wilderness of Dreaming.* Delacorte Press, 1996.

Bowra, C.M. *Classical Greece.* Time-Life Books, 1965.

Brodkey, J.H. "Passage into Non-existence," *Independent on Sunday Magazine,* London, 11 February, 1996.

Buber, Martin. *I and Thou,* trans. Walter Kaufman. T&T Clark, 1970.

Bunt, L. *Music Therapy: An Art Beyond Words.* Routledge, 1994.

Callahan, Daniel. *The Troubled Dream of Life.* Touchstone, 1993.

Callanan, Maggie and Keely, Patricia. *Final Gifts.* Bantam, 1993.

Campbell, Joseph. *Oriental Mythology: The Masks of God.* Arkana, 1991.

Cassell, Eric. *The Nature of Suffering and the Goals of Medicine.* Oxford University Press, 1991.

Charitonidou, Angeliki. *Epidauros.* Clio Editions, 1978.

Chodorow, J. *Dance Therapy and Depth Psychology: The Moving Imagination.* Routledge, 1991.

Comte, F. *Chambers Compact Reference: Mythology.* W&R Chambers, 1991.

Connell, C. *Something Understood: Art Therapy and Cancer Care.* Wrexham Publications, 1998.

Conrad, L., Neve, M., Nutton, V., Porter, R., and Wear, A. *The Western Medical Tradition.* Cambridge University Press, 1995.

Corbett, Lionel. *The Religious Function of the Psyche.* Routledge, 1996.

du Boulay, Shirley. *Cicely Saunders.* Hodder and Stoughton, 1984.

De Hennezel, Marie. *Intimate Death: How the Dying Teach Us to Live.* Little, Brown, 1997.

Duff, Kay. *The Alchemy of Illness.* Bell Tower, 1993.

Edelstein, Emma and Edelstein, Ludwig. *Asclepius: A Collection and Interpretation of the Testimonies,* Vols I and II. Johns Hopkins University Press, 1945.

Edelstein, Ludwig. "The Hippocratic Oath: Text, Translation and Interpretation," in *Ancient Medicine.* Johns Hopkins University Press, 1967.

———— . "Greek Medicine in its Relation to Religion and Medicine," in *Ancient Medicine.* Johns Hopkins University Press, 1967.

Edinger, Edward. *Ego and Archetype.* Shambhala, 1972.

Eliade, Mircea. *Shamanism: Archaic Techniques of Ecstasy.* Arkana, 1989.

Eliot, T.S. *Collected Poems 1909-1962.* Faber & Faber, 1963.

Farsides, C. and Garrard, E. "Resource Allocation in Palliative Care," in *New Themes in Palliative Care,* ed. D. Clark, J. Hockley, and S. Ahmedzai. Open University Press, 1997.

Fiefel, H. "Functions of Attitudes Towards Death," in *Death and Dying: Attitudes of Patients and Doctors.* Group for the Advancement of Psychiatry, 1965.

Field Guide to the Trees and Shrubs of Britain. Reader's Digest, 1981.

Fordham, Michael. *Countertransference: Explorations into the Self.* Academic Press, 1985.

Fox, Matthew, ed. *Meditations with Meister Ekhart.* Bear & Co, 1983.

Frankl, Viktor. *The Doctor and the Soul,* 2nd expanded edition. Pelican Books, 1973.

Freud, S. *The Interpretation of Dreams.* Penguin, 1976.

Graves, R. *The Greek Myths.* Penguin, 1960.

Groesbeck, C. Jess. "The Archetypal Image of the Wounded Healer," *Journal of Analytical Psychology* 20, 129, 1975.

Guggenbühl-Craig, Adolf. *Power in the Helping Professions.* Spring Publications, 1971.

Halifax, J. *Shaman: The Wounded Healer.* Thames and Hudson, 1982.

Hamilton, Mary. *Incubation or the Cure of Disease in Pagan Temples and Christian Churches.* Simpkin, Marshall, Hamilton, Kent & Co., 1906.

Heaney, Marie. *Over Nine Waves: A Book of Irish Legends.* Faber & Faber, 1994.

Hillman, James. *Suicide and the Soul.* Spring Publications, 1965.

——— . *Re-visioning Psychology.* Harper and Row, 1975.

——— . *The Dream and the Underworld.* Harper and Row, 1979.

——— . *Archetypal Psychology — A Brief Account.* Spring Publications, 1983.

——— . *Anima: An Anatomy of a Personified Notion.* Spring Publications, 1985.

——— and McLean, Margot. *Dream Animals.* Chronicle Books, 1997.

Hollister Wheelwright, Jane. *The Death of a Woman.* St. Martin's Press, 1981.

International Association for the Study of Pain Subcommittee on Taxonomy. "Pain Terms: A List with Definitions and Notes on Usage," *Pain* 8, 1980.

Johnson, D.F. and Grand, I.J. *The Body in Psychotherapy.* North Atlantic Books, 1998.

Jung, Carl G. *Psychological Reflections: A New Anthology of His Writings,* selected and edited by Jolande Jacobi. Routledge & Kegan Paul, 1971.

——— . *The Collected Works of C.G. Jung.* 2nd edition, trans. R.F.C. Hull, ed. by H. Read, M. Fordham, G. Adler and W. McGuire. (Princeton University Press, 1966-1970.

——— . *Memories, Dreams, Reflections.* UK: Flamingo, 1983.

Karcher, Stephen. *The I Ching.* Element, 1995.

Kasas, S. and Struckmann, R. *Important Medical Centres in Antiquity: Epidauros and Corinth.* Editions Kasas, 1990.

Kearney, Michael. "Palliative Medicine: Just Another Specialty?" *Palliative Medicine* 6(1), 1992.

——— . *Mortally Wounded: Stories of Soul Pain, Death and Healing.* Marino, 1996.

Kerenyi, Carl. *The Gods of the Greeks.* Thames and Hudson, 1951.

——— . *Asklepios: Archetypal Image of the Physician's Existence.* Pantheon, 1959.

——— . *Eleusis—Archetypal Image of Mother and Daughter,* trans. Ralph Manheim. Princeton University Press, 1967.

————. *Hermes: Guide of Souls.* Spring Publications, 1992.

Kreinheder, Albert. *Body and Soul: The Other Side of Illness.* Inner City Books, 1991.

Kugler, Paul. "Psychic Imaging: A Bridge Between Subject and Object," in *The Cambridge Companion to Jung.* Cambridge University Press, 1997.

Lawrence, D.H. *Complete Poems.* Penguin, 1993.

Lee, C., ed. *Lonely Waters: Proceedings of the International Conference on Music Therapy in Palliative Care.* Sobell Publications, 1995.

Lewis, C.S. *A Grief Observed.* Faber & Faber, 1961.

Lloyd, G.E.R., ed. *Hippocratic Writings.* Penguin, 1978.

Lopez, Barry. *The Rediscovery of North America.* Vintage, 1992.

Machtiger, H.G. "Countertransference/Transference," in *Jungian Analysis,* ed. M. Stein. Shambhala, 1985.

Marshall, Ian and Zohar, Danah. *Who's Afraid of Schrödinger's Cat?* Bloomsbury, 1997.

Martin, Peter. *The Experiment in Depth.* Routledge & Kegan Paul, 1955.

Meier, Carl, ed. *A Testament to the Wilderness.* Daimon, 1985.

————. *Healing Dream and Ritual.* Daimon, 1989.

McCarthy Draper, Maureen. *The Alchemy of Music: Beauty, Sound, and Healing.* Riverhead, 2000.

Miller, Henry. *The Colossus of Maroussi.* New Directions, 1958.

Moore, T., ed. *The Essential James Hillman: A Blue Fire.* Routledge, 1990.

Muff, Janet. "From the Wings of Night: Dream Work with People Who Have Acquired Immunodeficiency Syndrome," *Holistic Nurse Practitioner* 10 (4), 1996.

Neidjie, Bill, Davis, Stephen, and Fox, Allan. *Australia's Kakadu Man: Bill Neidjie.* Resource Managers, 1986.

Nutton, Vivian. "Medicine in the Greek World, 800-50 B.C.E.", in *The Western Medical Tradition,* ed. Lawrence I. Conrad, Michael Neve, Vivian Nutton, Roy Porter, and Andrew Wear. Cambridge University Press, 1995.

Obholzer, A. and Roberts, V., eds. *The Unconscious at Work: Individual and Organizational Stress in the Human Services.* Routledge, 1994.

Oliver, Mary. *Dream Work.* Atlantic Monthly Press, 1986.

————. *New and Selected Poems.* Beacon Press, 1992.

————. *White Pine.* Harcourt Brace Horida, Orlando, & Company, 1994.

————. *Blue Pastures.* Beacon Press, 1995.

————. *West Wind.* Houghton Mifflin, 1997.

————. *Winter Hours.* Houghton Mifflin, 1999.

Ovid. *Metamorphosis,* trans. Mary Innes. Penguin, 1955.

Paris, Ginette. *Pagan Meditations.* Spring Publications, 1986.

————. *Pagan Grace.* Spring, 1990.

Pausanias. *Guide to Greece,* volumes 1 and 2. Penguin, 1971.

Perry, Christopher. "Transference and Countertransference," in *The Cambridge Companion to Jung,* ed. Polly Young-Eisendrath and Terence Dawson. Cambridge University Press, 1997.

Pratt, A. and Wood, M., eds. *Art Therapy in Palliative Care: The Creative Response.* Routledge, 1998.

Preki-Alexandri, Kalliope. *Eleusis.* Archaeological Receipts Fund, 1991.

Racker, Heinrich. "The Meanings of Countertransference," *Psychoanalytic Quarterly* 26, 1957.

Ramsey, Jay. *Alchemy: The Art of Transformation.* Thorsons, 1997.

———— ed. *Earth Ascending: An Anthology of Living Poetry.* Stride, 1997.

Reading, A. *Illness and Disease,* Medical Clinics of North America 61, 1977.

Reed, Henry. "Dream Incubation: A Reconstruction of a Ritual in Contemporary Form," *Journal of Humanistic Psychology* 13, 3, 1974.

Reinhart, M. *Chiron and the Healing Journey.* Arkana, 1989.

Rilke, Rainer Maria. *Letters to a Young Poet.* Norton, 1993.

————. *Selected Poems,* trans. J. B. Leishman. Penguin, 1964.

————. *Selected Poems,* trans. Robert Bly. Harper and Row, 1981.

Ritsema, Rudolf and Karcher, Stephen. *I Ching.* Element, 1994.

Roszak, T., Gomes, M.E., and Kanner, A.D., eds. *Ecopsychology: Restoring the Earth, Healing the Mind.* Sierra Club Books, 1995.

Ryecroft, Charles. *A Critical Dictionary of Psychoanalysis.* Penguin, 1983.

Ryley, N., ed. *The Forsaken Garden.* Quest Books, 1998.

Samuels, A., Shorter, B. and Plaut, F. A *Critical Dictionary of Jungian Analysis.* Routledge & Kegan Paul, 1986.

Samuels, Andrew. *Jung and the Post-Jungians.* Routledge & Kegan Paul, 1985.

Saunders, Cicely. *The Management of Terminal Disease.* Edward Arnold, 1978.

————. *The Management of Terminal Malignant Disease,* 2nd edition. Edward Arnold, 1984.

Schouten, J. *The Rod and Serpent of Asklepios,* trans. M.E. Hollander. Elsevier, 1967.

Schroder, Patricia J. "Recognising Transference and Countertransference," *Journal of Psychosocial Nursing* 23(2), 1985.

Schwartz-Salant, Nathan. *C. G. Jung: Jung on Alchemy.* Routledge, 1995.

Sedgwick, David. *The Wounded Healer: Countertransference from a Jungian Perspective.* Routledge, 1994.

Shapiro, Colin M. *ABC of Sleep Disorders.* BMJ Publishing Group, 1993.

Shelburne, W.A. "A Critique of James Hillman's Approach to the Dream," *Journal of Analytical Psychology* 29, 39, 1984.

Shelley, Percy Bysshe. *Selected Poetry.* Penguin, 1956.

Skafte, Diane. *Listening to the Oracle.* Harper, 1997.

Snyder, G. *The Practise of the Wild.* North Point Press, 1990.

Solomon, S., Greenberg, J., and Pyszczynski, T. "Terror Management Theory of Self-esteem," in *Handbook of Social and Clinical Psychology: The Health Perspective,* eds. C.R. Synder and D. Forsyth. Pergamon, 1991a.

———. "A Terror Management Theory of Social Behaviour: The Psychological Functions of Self-esteem and Cultural Worldviews," in *Advances in Experimental Social Psychology,* ed. M.P. Zanna. Academic Press, San Diego, 1991b.

Speck, Peter. "Working with Dying People," in *The Unconscious at Work: Individual and Organisational Stress in the Human Services,* ed. Anton Obholzer and Vega Zagier Roberts. Routledge, 1994.

———. "Unconscious Communications," *Palliative Medicine* 10, 273, 1996.

Stedeford, Averil. "Hospice: A Safe Place to Suffer?" *Palliative Medicine* 1, 74, 1987.

Stevens, Anthony. *Private Myths: Dreams and Dreaming.* Penguin, 1995.

———. *The Two Million-Year-Old Self.* Fromm International, 1997.

Sullivan, J.W.N. *Beethoven, His Spiritual Development.* Random House, 1960.

Teilhard de Chardin, Pierre, *Activation of Energy.* Collins, 1970.

Thomas, R.S. *Collected Poems 1945-1990.* Phoenix Giants, 1993.

Twycross, R. and Lack, S. *Symptom Control in Far Advanced Cancer: Pain Relief.* Pitman, 1983.

van der Post, Laurens. *Jung and the Story of Our Time.* Penguin, 1976.

von Franz, Marie-Louise. *On Dreams and Death: A Jungian Interpretation.* Shambhala, 1987.

——— and Fraser Boa. *The Way of the Dream.* Shambhala, 1994.

Wagoner, David. *Who Shall be the Sun.* Indiana University Press, 1978.

Wasson, G., Ruck, C. and Hoffman, A. *The Road to Eleusis: Unveiling the Secret of the Mysteries.* Harcourt Brace Jovanovich, 1978.

Wellwood, John. *Awakening the Heart.* New Science Library, 1983.

Whitmont, Edward C. *The Symbolic Quest: Basic Concepts of Analytical Psychology.* Princeton University Press, 1969.

Whitmont, E.C. and Perera, S.B. *Dreams, A Portal to the Source.* Routledge, 1989.

Wilber, Ken. *The Marriage of Sense and Soul: Integrating Science and Religion.* Random House, 1998.

Wilhelm, Richard. *I Ching or Book of Changes.* Arkana, 1989.

Woodman, Marion. *The Pregnant Virgin.* Inner City Books, 1985.

———. *Conscious Femininity.* Inner City Books, 1993.

——— and Elinor Dickson, *Dancing in the Flames: The Dark Goddess in the Transformation of Consciousness.* Gill & Macmillan, 1996.

World Health Organization. *Cancer Pain Relief and Palliative Care.* Technical Report Series 804, 1990.

Young-Eisendrath, Polly and Dawson, Terence, eds. *The Cambridge Companion to Jung.* Cambridge University Press, 1997.

Zohar, Danah. *The Quantum Self.* Flamingo, 1991.

Zohar, Danah and Marshall, Ian. *The Quantum Society.* Flamingo, 1994.

———. *Spiritual Intelligence.* Bloomsbury, 2000.

Index

Bold entries indicate pages with illustrations

A